Life's too short to live without cheesecake

Understanding your motivation (or lack of it) for weight loss

By Jo Sherring

© 2018

Life's too short to live without cheesecake by Jo Sherring

© 2018 by Jo Sherring. All rights reserved.

No part of this book may be reproduced in any written, electronic, recording, or photocopying without written permission of the publisher or author. The exception would be in the case of brief quotations embodied in the critical articles or reviews and pages where permission is specifically granted by the publisher or author.

Although every precaution has been taken to verify the accuracy of the information contained herein, the author and publisher assume no responsibility for any errors or omissions. No liability is assumed for damages that may result from the use of information contained within.

Photography and Graphic Design (including cover) by Amanda Newton, Anew Creative

Editor: Michael Lefcourt

Formatting:

ISBN:

Keywords: health, weight loss, weight management, self-acceptance, body image, motivation, change

Author Biography

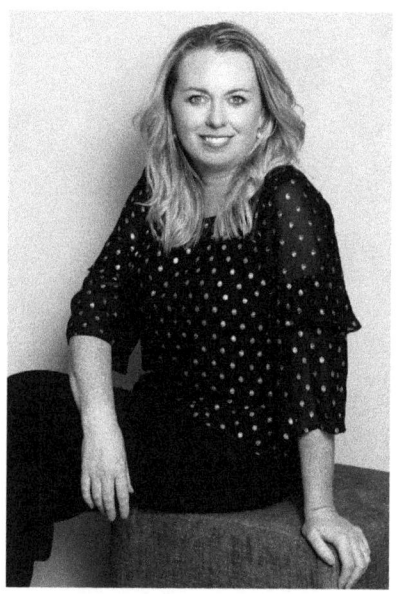

Jo Sherring is an occupational therapist who graduated from the University of Sydney in 1996 and spent twenty years working in the field of mental health. It was here that Jo developed a deep curiosity about human motivation and the factors that enabled people to make positive changes in their lives. Jo's reflections and research in this area led her to develop a number of tools to support better engagement of motivation. She has spent several years teaching health and disability staff about motivational concepts and helping clients to move past 'a lack of motivation'.

Jo lives in the tropical Australian city of Townsville with her husband and two children, where she continues to work in healthcare.

Life's too short to live without cheesecake is her first book.

For my daughter Maya,

who inspires me to make the world a better place.

For my son Evan,

who gives me the skills to do it.

And for my husband Peter,

who has the patience to let me try.

Contents

Section 1: Introduction to motivation 1

    Chapter 1: Buy a bigger dress 3

    Chapter 2: Not all motivation is equal 18

Section 2: Core motivational drivers 31

    Chapter 3: Personal values 32

    Chapter 4: Hope for life in general 45

    Chapter 5: Hope for weight management 56

    Chapter 6: Passion 66

    Chapter 7: Autonomy 76

    Chapter 8: Personality 89

    Chapter 9: Instinct 102

    Chapter 10: Intuition... 113

Section 3: Shallow motivational drivers 121

    Chapter 11: Attitudes and beliefs 122

    Chapter 12: Willpower 132

Chapter 13: Goals 144

Chapter 14: Habits 154

Chapter 15: Creating a new relationship with
your motivation 166

Chapter 16: Working with the motivation you have 175

Chapter 17: Questions you may have 193

Chapter 18: Tess and the dress 205

Acknowledgements 213

Interest Cards by Jo Sherring 215

Bibliography 217

Section 1

Introduction to motivation

CHAPTER 1

Buy a bigger dress

*'The shoe that fits one person pinches another;
There is no recipe for living that fits all cases'*

— Eleanor Roosevelt

'I am too big for my dress,' Tess complained. I sighed as she whinged yet again about how she had to lose weight. In the two years I had known this colleague and friend, I had seen her weight go up, go down, and go up again. She was frustrated with herself, and her weight was a regular topic of conversation between us.

The irony of course was Tess was a thin woman. 'I like to be fifty-eight kilograms,' she said. She was sixty-two kilograms. 'Why?' I asked her. 'It's just the weight I feel best at,' she answered. 'Why?' I asked again. 'I can fit into a size six or eight at that weight,' she replied. I inwardly groaned.

'You know the real answer to this problem?' I said to her. 'Go and buy a bigger dress.'

The conversation continued as I had expected, with Tess justifying why she needed to lose those few kilograms. But I knew the real problem—she was going to continue to do this up and down, guilt-driven, vanity-inspired behaviour for years to come—unless she understood herself better as a person, unless she realised motivation wasn't a simple choice, unless she stopped focusing on the size of her clothes and unless she embraced her natural motivational profile.

I had been in what felt like a million of these conversations over the years. Working in the female-dominated industry of healthcare, I had spent twenty years having lunch with women. I felt like I had seen and heard it all. I had seen women eat a lettuce leaf and take a pill, telling me this miracle diet was their new and easy way to lose kilograms without the need for exercise. I had seen women replace food with shakes and protein bars, only to give in two days later. I had watched weight go up and down, up and down, and up and down again over a period of years, while they went from various fads such as 'liver cleansing' to 'paleo' to 'clean food' to 'apple cider vinegar'. I had seen women pay large sums of money for diet programs only to eat tiny portions of pre-packaged food. I had seen some people refuse to put carbs near their mouth and then complain of their chronic constipation. I had heard the guilt, the theories, the crazy ideas and the stupid plans. I had seen people try to force down another salad for lunch, as excited by their meal as a trip to the dentist.

And I was done.

I couldn't watch the foolishness any longer. Tess's comments tipped me over the edge. I had to write a book about what I knew. Because I knew how motivation worked. And let me tell you one thing I knew for sure—motivation always made sense. There were reasons our motivation worked in a certain way. We were not deficient, we were not irresponsible and we were not 'unmotivated'. We just didn't know how our motivation worked. And for Tess's sake, and every other person I've ever heard complain about their weight, I had to do something about it.

My aim in writing this book is not to tell people how to 'get motivated'. My goal is to share some powerful knowledge to free people from guilt, frustration and 'battles'. I want people to understand how they actually work, to accept this, and to work in line with their motivation, so they never have to battle again.

I am not a thin person. I am not a fit person. I am not selling a weight loss plan. My weight goes up and down. My motivation for weight management goes up and down. And my life goes up and down. But I am not frustrated with my weight. I do not battle it because I know in the long run all those things are terrible for my motivation. In the long run, I am better focusing on the motivation I do have rather than the motivation I don't have. It is time to start talking about how we actually work rather than how we want to work, hope we work or believe we work. And that's why I told Tess to buy herself a bigger dress. She was 'battling' her weight, and any time we are 'battling', we are not in sync with our motivation.

Motivation is natural. It is a resource that we all have at our disposal. And we each have a unique motivational profile. This profile is the engine room of our motivation—it drives us, sustains us and energises us. Our motivation is not deficient. It is not a problem to be solved. It is a phenomenon to be understood. And once we have understood it, we can stop wasting our energy battling it and start putting our energy into working with it.

The reality is unless we have a very strong motivational profile for weight management, or are genetically programmed to be thin, it is likely in our current environment that we will struggle with weight management. How do I know that? Because when we have more than sixty per cent of our population struggling with weight, these people are behaving in their current environment in a completely and utterly normal manner. Sixty per cent of the population do not have extreme eating disorders, sixty per cent of the population do not disregard health advice, and sixty per cent of the population are not lazy. Sixty per cent of the population are doing exactly what is normal for their motivational profile in this current environment—which is making them fat. Our motivational profile is not something we can change, although it is something we can work with more effectively. However, this will only partially resolve the problem. The real focus for change needs to be on the environment. Relying on the motivation of individuals to solve the obesity crisis has failed, not because human beings are flawed but because human beings are human beings.

We each have a different motivational profile. Within this profile are strong motivational forces and weak motivational forces. These differences are an important part of our uniqueness and our human diversity. What this creates, though, are variations in motivational capacity for specific issues. Some people's profiles are aligned to engage with the aim of weight management, while others are not. While we all *want* to manage our weight, many of the motivational forces at our disposal are not something we chose or can even change. They are deeply embedded in our psyche and are present for our entire lives. Therefore, the desire to manage our weight is not enough to enable us to manage it. In fact, some psychologists believe that as little as twenty-five per cent of our behaviour is driven by deliberate intentions, leaving most of our behaviour to be driven by alternative forces.

The discussion in this book argues that people who are able to manage their weight in this current environment have a particular type of motivational profile. They have deep, subconscious forces in their nature that drive their behaviour for weight management. This is not a choice they have made, it is who they are within their individual nature. The flip-side of the discussion is that people, like myself, who struggle to manage their weight, have a different type of motivational profile that does not work in 'sync' with the goal of weight management. This does not mean we don't care about our weight, it just means it is not 'in our nature' to prioritise our weight. These 'core motivational drivers' are strong, sustainable and consistent influencers on our motivation and subsequent behaviour. These individual differences in motivational profiles were not a problem until we created an environment that was abundant in food and sedentary in nature. Those with a motivational profile that worked in sync with a weight management were able to adapt their behaviours to the new environment, not because they had better priorities or better motivation, but because their core drivers worked in alignment with the problem. The rest of us ended up feeling like failures. Battling our natures has been as successful as 'gay conversion therapy'- dismally ineffective.

Understanding our differences is key to understanding our motivation. The same people who have weak motivation for weight management will have strong motivation for other goals, which could be anything from raising money for a cause, saving abandoned animals, volunteering at the local school, or creating art and music. People with weak motivational forces for weight management are not weak people, it's just that their strengths and their strong motivational drivers sit in a different space.

By understanding how some of these differences work, my aim in writing this book is to help those with weak motivational drivers for weight management to not only understand themselves but to learn how to work with who they are more effectively when it comes to weight management. Ultimately, we all have a responsibility to take care of our health. We cannot ignore the dire consequences that can come from uncontrolled weight gain. As adults, we must continue to do what we can. But what we need to understand in more detail is our personal capacity and our personal limits. Not everyone has a motivational profile that supports getting up at five in the morning to exercise. But that doesn't mean we should quit! There are things that will suit your motivational profile better and will still have an impact.

A key part of that process is ditching the guilt and shame that comes along with weight struggles. As a result, though, this book may come with a message that's hard to swallow. You may never be thin in the current environment. This book may help you break unhealthy cycles and unhealthy approaches to weight, it may help you stop gaining weight, and, yes, you may even lose a little bit of weight. But working with your motivation in a healthy and realistic fashion may also mean accepting the fact that you will never again be the weight you were at twenty. I don't see this as a negative thing—I see this as a healthy acceptance of life's changes. What you don't want though is weight having major detrimental impacts on your health. You don't want to keep gaining weight over time. And you don't want to be a person who feels hopeless about the potential they *do* have to manage their weight within their capacity.

I didn't always know about motivation, and I have also used strategies that were unhelpful throughout my life. Learning about motivation has been a journey spanning twenty years, so let me share a little about this journey with you.

How did I learn about motivation?

I am an occupational therapist and I graduated from the University of Sydney in 1996. Occupational therapy is one of those obscure professions that is often misunderstood, so let me explain it in simple terms. Occupational therapy is based on the idea that people need to do activities and fulfil roles that are meaningful to them in order to experience health and wellbeing. A person sitting at home who is bored, lonely and feels their life holds little meaning would therefore be considered 'unhealthy' from this perspective. An occupational therapy viewpoint would be that this person lacks 'meaningful occupational roles'. As such, a therapist may support the person to improve their health and wellbeing, by helping them to connect and engage with things that brought them fulfilment, achievement and joy.

I worked as an occupational therapist in the field of mental health for twenty years in Australia. My aim was to help people with mental illness to engage in meaningful roles and activities to support their health. You might assume my clients were grateful to receive my help and support. Not necessarily! What I found was that many people I worked with were 'unmotivated'. While my aim was to help them engage in things to make their life better and more meaningful, there was often a reluctance from their side to actually make that happen!

Here I was, enthusiastic and ready to help, but I struggled to help clients get into a motivated space so they could achieve the things they said they wanted. I attempted to work in partnership with them and we would identify goals such as 'get a job', 'lose weight', 'make more friends', 'get fit', 'learn a hobby' or 'gain a qualification'. We would spend months, if not years, where I tried to support them to pursue these goals. Together we'd break the goals down into small 'realistic' steps, we'd set timeframes and we'd talk about the value of the goal. But ultimately, in many cases, these goals were never achieved. My clients genuinely seemed to want these changes, but they struggled to make any real progress, even with all my support, goal setting and strategies for success. I tried to be helpful, but, ultimately, I felt I spent a lot of wasted time trying to get people *motivated*.

At the time, I didn't comprehend how complex motivation was, and it was clear that those around me didn't either. I worked with psychiatrists, psychologists, nurses, social workers, general practitioners, employment officers, support workers and a range of other professionals. We were all highly trained, we were all extremely enthusiastic and we were all full of good intentions. But none of us could understand why these people seemed so stuck.

After a decade of working in a manner where I continually labelled people as 'unmotivated', I started to change my point of view. Instead of focusing on the people who didn't achieve their goals, I started to notice the few people who did. I began to identify what was happening within them, and around them, that supported the change process towards their goals. And I started to recognise that there were some key things happening in these situations. In particular, I paid attention when people went from years of being 'stuck' to suddenly having a spark of energy that drove them towards progress. Almost subconsciously, I began to understand how motivation actually worked. And I also started to notice that many of the strategies, and much of the thinking we were using around motivation, was not only unhelpful but potentially damaging to the person's motivational process.

It would take a few more years to articulate these thoughts in a way that made sense. One day I was running a training session with staff who worked in the disability field. They expressed their frustration that many of their clients 'lacked motivation'. During the discussion that followed, I wrote a list on the whiteboard of the things I felt influenced motivation. This is what that list looked like:

1. People will only be motivated if they are interested in the change.

2. People will only be motivated if they have hope that the change is possible.

3. People will only be motivated if they have a clear vision of what this change looks like.

4. People will only be motivated if they believe they have the capacity to create the change.

5. People will only be motivated if they value the difference the change will make to their lives.

6. People will only be motivated if their intuition tells them this change feels right, right now.

7. People will only be motivated if they feel in control of the process to create the change.

8. People will only be motivated if they are prepared to tolerate the discomfort the change process will bring.

In writing this list, I felt it was the first time I had clearly articulated motivation for other people. So, I started using this list to assist my colleagues in the health and disability industry to reflect on motivation and called it the 'Motivation to Create Change Theory' (MCC). Over the next few years I would investigate what the research said about motivation to find out if my 'hunch' was supported by research. MCC helped me to pull together ideas and research that came from various fields of psychology and social science, and as I studied the science behind motivation I found some amazing and compelling information. Not only was my hunch on track, I discovered more to motivation than I could have anticipated. The combination of my experience as a clinician, my personal reflections from MCC and the findings of this research now form the basis of my understanding for motivation.

While the MCC list still has some merit and may be useful in certain situations, I will not be using this format to explain motivation in the book. I felt it was better to use an approach that more effectively explains strong motivational forces against weak motivational forces, which I call the 'Onion Theory'. I will explain how this works in chapter 2.

Motivation and weight management

As I learnt more about human motivation over the years I found myself developing a deep frustration about the overly simplistic messages I saw on the topic of weight management. It seemed the world was determined to make us all feel bad about ourselves, which is in fact a terrible motivator. While well intentioned, the information in my opinion was unhelpful and sometimes just completely inaccurate or obnoxious. 'Follow our plan and become the real you.' Are you suggesting people need to be thin to be 'real'? Or one of my personal favourites, 'Get up an hour earlier every day and exercise.' Are we telling this to mothers who have been up all night with babies—those who are chronically sleep deprived and exhausted? Does anyone remember the research linking better sleep to better weight management?

One that would pop up in social media every now and then was a picture of an extremely thin woman in a bikini and written above her were the words 'No excuses!' I found this one particularly offensive. When I worked as a mental health clinician I saw young people put on twenty kilograms in six months after starting psychiatric medications that are well known for creating weight gain. No excuses? I had seen my friend Elizabeth survive fifteen years of a chaotic and at times abusive relationship, while keeping her three children safe. She eventually managed to leave, but with no money and little support to rebuild her life. One of the side effects of her survival was significant weight gain. Again, no excuses? The period when I gained the most weight, I was struggling with an increase in violent behaviour from my son, who has autism and an intellectual disability. I was dealing with daily hitting, scratching and hair pulling. Taking care of my own health was beyond my capacity at the time. Do we really say no excuses? 'No excuses' flippantly disregards the very real challenges people face in life. It is not always easy, or at the top of people's priority lists, to worry about their weight. Sometimes people are just busy surviving the day.

Even our well-intentioned health professionals get this wrong at times. When my friend Elizabeth went to a new general practitioner (GP) with some health concerns, the GP said to her, 'Well you are obese'. Only just starting to recover from the trauma of her experiences, my friend had spent the previous twelve months getting work, finding accommodation for her family, settling the children into new schools, gaining some financial stability and attending therapy with her kids to deal with the emotional fallout of what they had been through. She now wanted to focus on some of her broader health issues. This comment from the GP was shaming. It insinuated that 'This is all your fault' with no recognition of what she had been through or how far she had come. Did the GP really think my friend didn't know her weight was a problem? Elizabeth left feeling judged, not inspired to lose weight.

Weight gain always has a story behind it. My friend Elizabeth's story is of course relevant to her weight issues. Other people's stories may not be as dramatic or even obvious, but there will always be a valid story for every person who has weight issues. I sometimes think about my sister, who is a dietitian and works as a lecturer and researcher at a university. With all her knowledge, even she struggles to maintain her weight. She has three kids and works fulltime. Her husband works in a job where he travels frequently. She spends her afternoons and weekends running around to and from her kids' activities, and her evenings are spent marking papers or reading research reports. None of her three kids have been good sleepers—she hasn't seen a full night's sleep in fourteen years! On top of this, add washing, ironing, shopping, cooking, cleaning and everything else a woman has to manage. She knows everything there is to know about food and weight; in fact, she teaches it. But she still struggles with her weight. She has a story, and it is a story many people can relate to—a story of exhaustion and lack of time and competing priorities. We can't just 'educate' people out of being overweight. We need to truly understand what is happening within the story of their lives. Motivation for weight management is a complex issue, and it requires complex reflection of the issues at hand, not catch phrases such as 'No excuses!'

Many weight management messages in the world come to us from the people who are **not** struggling with their weight—the thin, fit people of the world. Some of these people think that if they can do it, then you can do it too. They are the ones telling us to get up an hour earlier, to cut out carbs, to set goals and have 'better' priorities. They post pictures of their perfect, toned bodies. They tell us about their twelve-week programs, their seven minutes of exercise a day, their cleansing juices and their metabolism-boosting diets. And the irony is, I think most of these people genuinely want to be helpful. But there is a big problem. They are different to those of us who struggle with weight management. They are the ones with the motivational drivers coming from the seventy-five per cent subconscious space. They have a motivational profile that supports *this* specific weight management goal. And this is not something they have any control over.

I have nothing against the thin and fit people of the world—they are just being themselves after all. But what I do have a problem with is when these people assume they have the answers to weight management simply because they are fit and thin. Again, it's not their fault that they think this; they have had these messages reinforced by the community over the past several decades. They think it is because of what they do that they are thin and fit, but in fact the reality is a little bit more complex. They are in fact thin and fit because of who they are. What's the difference you may ask? What they do is driven by the seventy-five per cent of their motivational forces. It is about who they are at their 'core'. And at their core, they have a certain set of motivational drivers that enable their behaviour, resulting in them being thin and fit.

At this point, you may wish that you had these same motivational drivers sitting in your subconscious. Before you long for something you don't have though, let me share an important point. To have strong motivational drivers for weight management you would have to lose strong motivational drivers for something else. And usually what we have strong motivational drivers for is in fact more important to us. We are literally pulled away from some things and towards others at a subconscious level. How often do you think that Mother Theresa worried about the size of her thighs? I very much doubt it came to her mind at all. What did she contribute to the world by not focusing on her weight though? Or what about Oprah? Did anyone like Oprah less, or value what she did in the world less, when she gained weight? Was she less intelligent, or less generous, because she was heavier on the scales? No, she was as popular as ever! When you think about Oprah, you don't define her by the size of her arse, you define her by the size of her heart. Mother Theresa and Oprah have motivational profiles as givers, not motivational profiles for weight management. Their deep motivational drivers are about other people. And these sit within a space so embedded within their psyche that they are unable to fight them. They would prioritise giving to others over their own personal achievement whether they wanted to or not. *It is who they are at their core.*

People who are strongly motivated to manage their weight are often the opposite. That doesn't make them bad people, it just makes them *different* people. They can still deeply care about others; however, when they prioritise their time and their energy, they are *more likely* to be motivationally driven towards their own success. When it comes to core motivational drivers, opposites exist. As a result, people who tend to be givers also tend to be people who struggle with their weight. The strong motivation to give is opposite to the strong motivation for achievement or personal image. It is not possible to have both at the same strength. The strength of these drivers and their opposites is established before we reach adulthood. It is not something we choose, it is something we absorb and develop in our childhood. This absorption process happens due to a combination of factors, and eventually supports one of our strongest motivational drivers: our values. We will explore values and how these opposites work in chapter 3, but first, there are some other things about motivation to understand.

CHAPTER 2

Not all motivation is equal

'I did then what I knew how to do. Now that I know better, I do better'

— Maya Angelou

When it comes to motivation, there are some things that have strong 'motivational pull' and others that are weaker. When I observe people around me trying to manage their weight, it seems to me they rely on their weaker motivational forces rather than their stronger ones. The weaker forces are useful tools at our disposal, but they are only effective if they work in line with the stronger motivational forces within us. These forces can only have so much impact on the overall aim of weight management. That is why we call weight management a 'battle', because that is exactly what it feels like!

The battle happens when we put weak motivational forces against much stronger motivational forces. Eventually our weak forces 'run out of steam'. People are able to sustain their effort or 'battle' for a period of time, but eventually the stronger forces gain the upper hand. The negative impact of this process is that people feel like failures. How often do you see people post on social media, 'Look, I've gained ten kilos'? The slow return of weight after a diet is never a source of celebration; in fact, it is often a source of deep shame. This cycle is incredibly important to understand, because it has long-term implications for our stronger motivational forces.

The first concept to grasp is this: do not put strong motivational forces into conflict with weak motivational forces. It is not logical and leads to inevitable failure and despair. It is like putting a ten-year-old girl into a tug of war against a twenty-year-old man and expecting her to win. This is the scenario that most diets place us in. While we may be able to put up a good fight, eventually fatigue and exhaustion from the battle set in. Long-term battles are not sustainable from a psychological perspective.

I may as well say this right now: never diet again. Diets are illogical and set us up to fail. We may gain a short-term outcome but we damage motivational forces required for long-term sustainable change. This potentially puts us in a position of even greater weight gain. I know it's tough to give up the idea of a quick fix, but this book is about the long-term outcome of health. If you just want to lose weight for a wedding or a high school reunion, please go and buy another book!

The Onion Theory

To ensure the strong and weak motivational forces are easier to understand, I am going to use a visual concept I call the 'Onion

Theory'. In the animated movie Shrek, the ogre tells the donkey he is made up of layers', like an onion. He was suggesting there was a deeper side of him that people didn't always see. In fact, this analogy is spot-on for all of us. Obviously, this is just a way of describing concepts, but there are some psychologists who have written and researched the idea of psychological layers. Here are some of the key points for the Onion Theory:

- With an onion, there are layers that sit deep in the 'core' and then there are other layers that are surface or 'superficial'. The deep layers contain the strong motivational forces. The shallow or 'superficial' layers contain the weak motivational forces.

- The core motivational forces are different from the superficial motivational forces. The core forces are stable and rarely change over a person's lifetime. The superficial forces change more easily and can be swayed by new information or attitudes.

- The core motivational forces sustain behaviour in the long term. The superficial motivational forces have less impact and often only influence short-term behaviour.

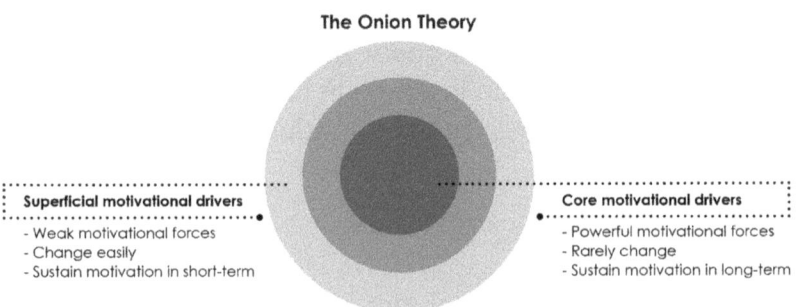

The Onion Theory

Superficial motivational drivers
- Weak motivational forces
- Change easily
- Sustain motivation in short-term

Core motivational drivers
- Powerful motivational forces
- Rarely change
- Sustain motivation in long-term

The forces at the core are the engine room of our motivation. The core is where our real motivational forces or drive comes from. The superficial layers can improve performance of the engine, but they are not the source of the motivational forces we experience. That comes from deep within us.

The core motivational forces sit in our subconscious. We are less aware of their influence on our behaviour. They also drive our motivation across different contexts or environments. For example, they influence us at home, at work, at school, during our hobbies, our travel and all other activities. They are very consistent.

Superficial motivational forces tend to sit in our conscious thoughts. They only influence us in some contexts and can be very inconsistent. For example, it is not uncommon for people to 'start a diet' every Monday. Often by Wednesday they are sitting in a restaurant eating double cheese pizza. The superficial motivational forces can be influenced easily by our mood on the day, hunger or just seeing something we like to eat!

In this book I will bring some of these deeper motivational forces into conscious focus. When we know what they are and how they work, we can make more informed decisions. This will include how to use our superficial forces in line with our core forces. That is how we get the most out of our motivation! Remember, we're not creating motivation here, we are working with the motivation we already have. It is a very different way of thinking. The aim is to harness our motivation and not set ourselves up in a battle with our own nature.

Another important part of the layer concept is to understand intrinsic and extrinsic motivation and how they interact with each other.

Intrinsic and extrinsic motivation

My daughter has loved creative activities from when she was very young. At the age of five she announced to me, 'I want to be an artist when I grow up!' I took this about as seriously as you would from a five-year-old but wanted to know more about why she enjoyed art. So, I asked her, 'What is it you like about art?' She thought about it for a moment and replied 'I don't know why I like it. I was just born loving it.' This is a perfect description of intrinsic motivation. Something we were just 'born loving'.

Intrinsic motivation comes from the things that are inherently important to us as individuals. We do them simply for the inner feeling of joy or accomplishment. It is almost 'instinctive' in nature. I love watching children play, as you can see their intrinsic natures early in their development. You can pick out the children who love music, the ones who love a physical challenge, those who enjoy social contact, the ones who like to learn, and others who want to explore. It is as if they are still 'pure' in their motivational drivers. The world around them has not yet become a strong enough influence on their motivation to confuse their true natures.

Extrinsic motivation comes from outside of us. The classic example is an animal receiving a food reward when they are being trained. I have never seen a seal or dolphin perform without being given a piece of fish as a reward. There's a good reason for that. Research shows the behaviour stops once the reward stops. With humans, the most obvious extrinsic driver is the money we earn from going to work. If they stopped paying us, would we still turn up? I don't think so!

There are many other extrinsic motivators that influence our behaviour though. For example, the approval of other people is often an influence on what we do and why. Our parents might expect us to do things, our teachers might encourage us to do things, and our culture might influence us to do things. While children are born with an innate desire to partake in activities, they quickly learn the things for which they get approval from their parents. Tommy may be an enthusiastic musician at first, but when he realises that Dad wants to play with him when he does sport, he may redirect his energy towards these activities.

Extrinsic motivation is very relevant to the discussion about weight management. Tess complained to me that she had gained weight. When I asked her why she wanted to lose weight, she at first seemed to be intrinsically motivated: 'I feel better at that weight'. But when I dug deeper and asked her why that was the case, she said, 'I can fit into a size six or eight at that weight'. This revealed an extrinsic motivational driver. Why was it important to be a certain size in clothes? The answer was actually about cultural expectations of a 'good' size. Wanting to be a certain size in clothes is *not* an intrinsic motivator, even though my friend 'wanted it'. When explored further, the positive gain for her would have been from social endorsement, which is an element of an extrinsic reward system.

The providing of advice and recommendations to patients by health professionals is also an extrinsic motivational force. What may be defined as encouragement can in fact be a form of external pressure to comply (even when that is health related). For example, the body mass index, which identifies people as fitting into categories such as 'overweight' or 'obese', is an extrinsic motivational driver. These categories are aimed at 'motivating' us to move into a healthier category. But they are in fact a weak form of motivation.

Social expectations and standards are developed through a process called social constructionism. Over time as a community, we receive the same messages so many times that we translate these into a 'reality'. Despite the repetition, these messages only represent a belief, but a belief created and shared by so many people that we don't see it as anything other than fact.

If you are old enough, you may remember the era in which the community defined dietary fat as bad. It was socially constructed by society as a 'fact'. As a result, the supermarket shelves were swamped with low-fat items to meet the desire we had for low-fat foods. My sister the dietitian was one of the few people I heard warning against this low-fat craze. She insisted that fats held essential nutrients that were important in our diets. And of course, the community now recognises that too. The community opinion has now swung more towards a high-protein diet, although, let me tell you, the dietitians don't think this plan is good either!

As cultures, we develop 'realities' based on what the community says. At this point, our culture has developed a reality in which 'fat people are unhealthy'. Is it really a fact though? While people who are overweight are more likely to have health problems, there are actually people who are overweight who are also healthy. We've all heard that the Mediterranean diet is good for us. It is high in legumes, vegetables, seafood and olive oil. But the people of the Mediterranean are not necessarily thin. And so, this shows that we need to be careful in jumping to too many conclusions. Is our aim really thinness or is it actually health? If it's health, the number on the scale has less importance than our current social construct suggests.

In our culture, we associate weight with health. Obviously, thin people can also be extremely unhealthy. I know thin people who've had cardiac bypass surgery. I know thin people who live on takeaway food. I know thin people who consume two or three times the recommended intake of alcohol a day. I know thin people who can't walk up a flight of stairs without puffing. Not all thin people are healthy. But we assume they are, or at least superficially. Just to prove my point, I looked up 'healthy people' on Google Images. And what I saw confirmed everything I believe the community thinks about health: thin people were exercising and eating salad. This is a very one-dimensional perspective of health. I kept scrolling through the images until I eventually found someone who wasn't really thin. It was a picture of a stomach with a tape measure around it. It suggests a prototype for health, which is a problem, because the focus is inadvertently primarily on weight, when we know that health is influenced by a huge number of factors. Instead of wondering if we can assist overweight people to be healthier, we've tended to focus primarily on overweight people getting thinner.

Losing weight *may* help overweight people improve their health, but it is certainly not the only pathway or the only measure of a healthy person. Motivationally, this creates an enormous social pressure to fit within a certain weight range. And this is an *extrinsic motivator*. While this motivator has been communicated with the best of intentions, it may be causing a real problem.

And this is where things get complicated. Extrinsic motivators actually decrease intrinsic motivation in pursuing a goal. Sounds ridiculous, right? No. There is research dating back to the 1960s that verifies this fact. When we use an extrinsic motivator to try and get a person to change, doing so will decrease their intrinsic motivation for that activity.

And yet, it is our *intrinsic* motivation that holds the real power when it comes to what we do. Research demonstrates that when we are driven by internal motivators, we are able to sustain behaviours, push through challenges and problems, and have far more successful outcomes. Our intrinsic motivators are our strong motivational drivers. Our strong motivational drivers make up our motivational engine room.

On the other hand, our extrinsic motivators are fickle. They work for short periods but tend to fail in the long term because we have created a battle. It is a scenario setting people up to fail. It is not about people being 'unmotivated', but about people being completely normal.

There are two types of people maintaining their weight in the current environment:

1. Naturally thin people who can eat anything and do no exercise. Some of my best friends fall into this category. I love them, but it is not motivation keeping them thin—it is genetics.

2. The people who are functioning from core motivational drivers to sustain their weight. These people will have a particular motivational profile that supports weight management.

And then there's the rest of us, struggling along to maintain our weight in a world that is determined to keep us eating and sedentary.

If we genuinely want to harness the motivation we have, we need to function from our intrinsic motivators. If we try and function from extrinsic motivators, we in fact decrease the effect of our intrinsic forces. The consistent forces. The strong forces. The reliable forces.

The world though is trying to use extrinsic forces to get us to change: the health messages, the pictures of fit people, the advice from doctors, and the media reports telling us how fat we are. All these ruin our greatest motivational powerhouse: our intrinsic motivation for weight management.

However, getting to the heart of our intrinsic motivation involves getting to the heart of who we are as people. Just because we 'want' something doesn't mean we want it because of intrinsic forces. Psychologists refer to this as 'locus of causality'. If the reason we want it comes from a 'cause' outside of ourselves, the want is extrinsic in nature. Therefore, fitting into a size eight pair of jeans is extrinsic. Getting a 'revenge body' to make an ex-boyfriend jealous is extrinsic. Losing weight to look better in wedding photos in extrinsic.

Intrinsic forces are about who you are as a person and what naturally drives you. These forces are about joy, and health and wellbeing.

The rest of the book will take you through several steps:

1. Learning about some of your core motivational drivers and how they work

2. Learning about the weak motivational drivers we often use to try and manage weight

3. Understanding how to stop battles and how to work in alignment with your motivation.

Motivation is obviously more complex than two layers. In fact, motivation is more complex than the components listed in this book. My aim though is to give you enough information to progress your thinking from 'there is something wrong with my motivation' to 'my motivation is normal and a part of who I am'. I am hoping this will be enough to help you work in alignment with who you are, free you from negativity and allow you to take steps that actually work for health in the long term.

The chapters in sections two and three of the book will each cover a different motivational concept. This makes the chapters easy to read and understand, but of course motivation at any point is determined by the combined forces of these motivational drivers and how they interact with one another. You therefore cannot consider the motivational impact of something such as 'personality' in isolation from other factors such as 'hope'. The book therefore needs to be considered as a whole, not as separate chapters in isolation.

Section two of the book covers core motivational drivers and is separated into the following chapters:

- Personal values
- Hope for life in general
- Hope for weight management

- Passion
- Autonomy
- Personality
- Instinct
- Intuition

Section three of the book then focuses on shallower motivational drivers, covering the following:

- Attitudes and beliefs
- Willpower
- Goals
- Habits

Finally, in section four, I discuss how you can identify your core motivational drivers and use strategies that work with these rather than against them. I also answer questions you may have about moving forward such as 'Should I weigh myself regularly?' and 'Should I go to a personal trainer?' I then touch on what we could consider doing as a society to reduce the environmental pressure attacking our weight and our ability to manage it successfully. I share many of my own personal challenges through the book and discuss stories from a number of people I know. These people, in some instances, have been identified by their real names, but in other instances, not. But they were all happy to allow their stories to be used so I could talk about the 'normal' in human beings and how gloriously diverse and imperfect we really are!

SECTION 2

CORE MOTIVATIONAL DRIVERS

CHAPTER 3

Personal values

*'Before you tell your life what truths and values you have decided to live up to,
let your life tell you what truths you embody, what values you represent'*

— Parker Palmer

I once told a friend who was single to do a test within the first month of dating any new man. I suggested she play a game of Monopoly. 'You can tell a lot about a person from the way they play Monopoly,' I told her. She laughed, but I swore by this technique as a way of getting to the 'heart' of who a man really was, telling her about an ex I had who turned into a maniac the minute a board game came out. He valued winning over any friendship and would show a nasty streak normally hidden by social protocol. It was a warning sign I wish I had paid more attention to earlier.

Values are broad goals that influence our behaviour across different contexts and situations in our lives. An achievement-oriented person will be achievement oriented at work, in sport, while studying, at home and even during a game of Monopoly! Our values are strong and consistent influencers of our behaviour and motivation. They develop early in our lives and are set by the time we reach adulthood. They rarely change after that time. We do not choose our values. The process of 'obtaining' values happens subconsciously and is influenced by many factors, such as our personality, our life experiences, the era in which we were born, our family, our education and our culture. All these variables are absorbed to varying degrees by our subconscious. This happens in an individualised manner that is not clearly understood—even people in the same family can have quite different values.

In everyday conversation, we tend to identify the following as values: integrity, honesty, compassion and respect. However, these concepts actually sit in a shallower space in our psyche and are a part of our beliefs and attitudes. There are an infinite number of beliefs and attitudes but a limited number of personal human values. We all hold varying degrees of each of these values in our personal profiles. What differs between individuals is the strength of each one of them. Shalom Schwartz and his colleagues from the University of Jerusalem spent years researching the concept. As a result, we now have an idea about how values function and how they influence behaviour. We also have a better understanding of how each relates to one another.

I mentioned in the first chapter that values have opposites. Professor Schwartz and his colleagues determined this by using mathematical equations to 'map' human values. Values work together as a system rather than as individual concepts. Therefore, what actually influences our behaviour is how these values work together as a group. Professor Schwartz describes them as functioning in a similar manner to a colour wheel: the values situated close together are similar in nature, while those on the opposite side of the wheel are opposite in nature. It is far easier to understand this by looking at the following diagram:

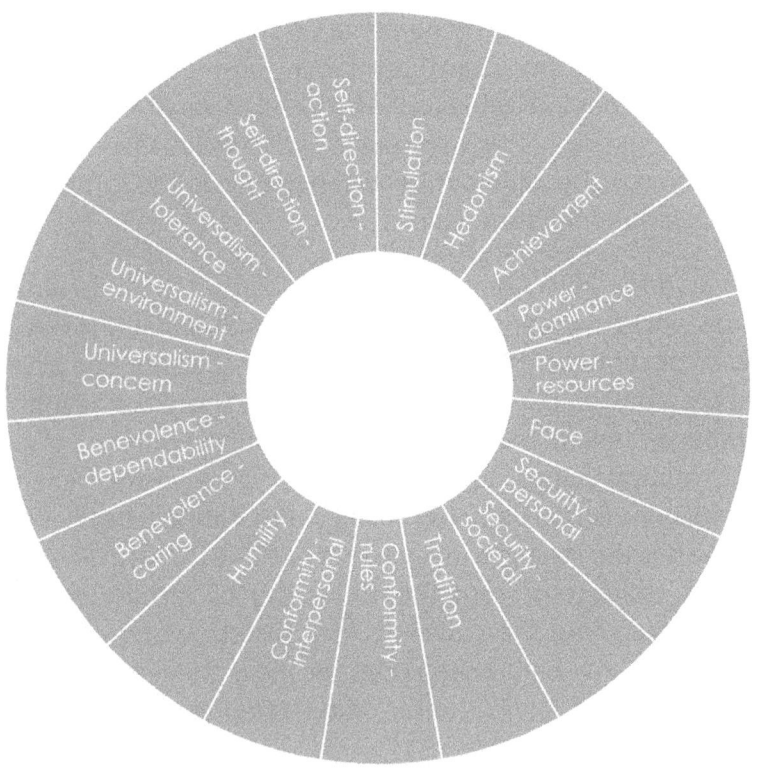

Adapted from Schwartz et al. (2012), 'Refining the theory of basic individual values', *Journal of Personality and Social Psychology*, vol. 103, no. 4, 663–688.

I have listed brief descriptions of each of these values in the following table:

Value	Explanation
Stimulation	Enjoying new experiences, challenges, learning and adventures
Hedonism	Focus on pleasure and fun
Achievement	Wanting success in socially endorsed areas
Power—dominance	Desiring power over other people or groups
Power—resources	A drive towards power from money or possessions
Face	Personal image being of importance
Security—personal	Wanting security for yourself and one's immediate social group
Security—societal	Desiring the security of one's community or country
Tradition	Cultural norms, traditions or standards of a social group being important
Conformity—rules	Conforming to social rules and laws
Conformity—interpersonal	Wanting to meet other people's expectations and social norms
Humility	Seeing oneself as part of something bigger
Benevolence—caring	Focusing on the care of people in your social group
Benevolence—dependability	Importance on other people being able to rely upon you
Universalism—concern	Caring for all people in the world, known and unknown
Universalism—environment	Focusing on issues related to animals, nature and the environment
Universalism—tolerance	Accepting difference and wanting everyone to have the same rights
Self-direction—thought	A strong desire to think for oneself and have original thought
Self-direction—action	A drive to determine your own behaviour, actions and destiny

I have a values profile that makes it hard for me to manage my weight. This doesn't mean that it is impossible, but my values profile creates challenges. Like most people, I didn't have much of an idea about my values or what they 'looked like'. Having read about the idea of a colour wheel, I decided I needed to see what this 'pulling effect' looked like in a visual format.

Therefore, in a very unscientific manner, I came up with a set of questions that related to each of the values, and I wrote them on cards. I then rated each of my answers from 1 to 10 (10 being of very high value). I placed all the cards around a picture of the wheel, with the highest rating cards sitting closest to the wheel, and the weaker ones sitting further away. This photograph was the result of that exercise:

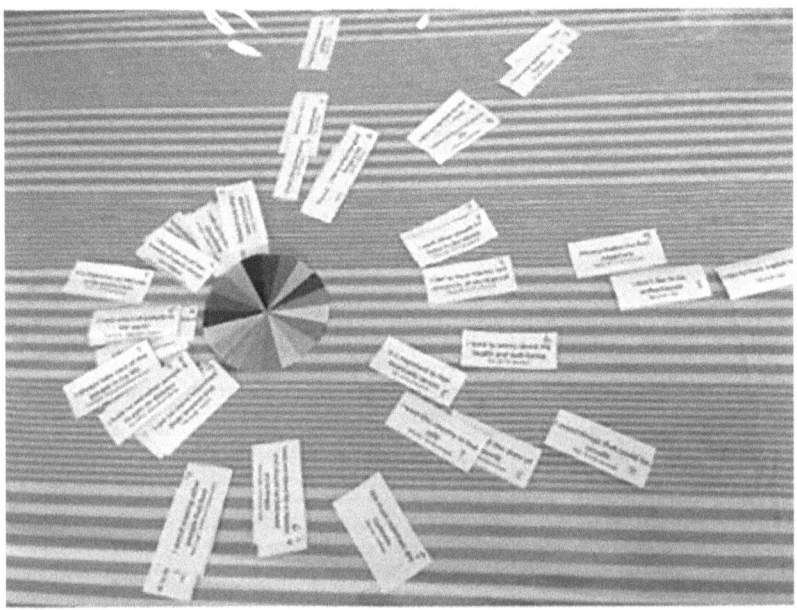

As you can clearly see from the photograph, I had a motivational pull to one side of the values wheel. The items of most importance to me were from the self-direction category, down the left-hand side to humility. Now please don't confuse this activity with science—this was just an activity I made up for myself one Sunday afternoon! But what happened to me as this image came together had a profound impact on me: it felt like the first time I had truly understood why I did things (or didn't do things). What this picture told me was that I am motivationally driven as a giver. What it also told me was that the combined values on the other side of the wheel were not strong enough to pull me away from being a giver. If this had been a tug of war, the giver side was always, always going to win.

What struck me as I saw my own values profile develop was a sense of not only understanding myself but also forgiving myself. I realised, perhaps for the first time, that I couldn't fight who I was. Battling my true nature was not only useless but completely illogical. No matter how much 'positive thinking' or 'goal setting' I did, I would inevitably be drawn back to my true nature as a giver. It was a blessed relief to realise at the age of forty that I could give up all the energy I had been expending trying to pull myself towards the other side of the wheel! Let's have a look at some of the things I have freed myself from as a result of understanding my values more effectively.

1. **Having a clean house**

A clean house is likely to be driven by the value of 'face' or perhaps even 'achievement'. A clean house is a socially condoned concept. If we believed what we saw in the media, people who have untidy houses are dysfunctional in some way. But no, actually, it is because *I am a giver* that I struggle to keep a tidy house. I am too busy changing the world (or just focusing on spending time with my children). This all sits within my 'giver' nature. Therefore, my house stays in a state of what I might call 'haphazard cleanliness'. It's kept in a tolerable state that is neither entirely clean or tidy, but not entirely chaotic or filthy. I am now okay with that, as I know that no matter how hard I try, how many label-makers I buy, or how many organisational tools I implement, my house is always going to be that way!

2. **Academic achievement**

There once was a time when I thought I needed to publish in academic, peer-reviewed journals to be credible. This idea was strongly encouraged by people around me, and was driven by the evidence-based, scientific world of health I had lived in for twenty or more years. I gave academic writing a half-hearted attempt but could never seem to 'motivate' myself to get it done. It felt like a laborious task that was expected of me, rather than something that brought me joy in and of itself.

Academic writing would have sat in an achievement values space. While I do achieve, and even enjoy it, *it is not my core motivational pull.* Achievement rated at about a seven or an eight out of ten. The items directly opposite rated at a nine or ten out of ten. So even though academic writing rated quite highly, when it came down to conflict between the two opposing sides, motivationally achievement would lose. And that was why I procrastinated with academic writing. It wasn't 'in my nature' to focus on it with true drive and determination. I was far more interested in storytelling than academia. I have now embraced this as who I am, not as a less valid form of expression or reflection.

3. Wanting to be skinny

I've been skinny. It was nice. I could go into any shop and buy most things and look reasonable in them. Skinniness was definitely rewarded and admired by the world around me. But was it deeply fulfilling, life altering and the core of who I was as a person? No. The work I have done through my job, my writing and teaching have been all these things though.

The reality is, while being skinny gives some social credit, it didn't do any of the things that are really important to me based on my values profile. Therefore, when I had to choose between spending time to write or to exercise (a choice I often faced), I had a tendency to choose writing. This wasn't always a conscious choice—I was just pulled in that direction in a stronger way. Being skinny wasn't important enough to me to pull me away from the other things that drove me as a human being. I no longer wonder why I can't 'get motivated' to lose weight.

I've made many other profound insights into why I do things from the values profile activity I completed. The longest I have ever stayed in one job was five years. I now see that this was driven by a need for stimulation and new learning. Once I felt I had gained competence and achievement in a job, I looked for new adventures and challenges. I had also left jobs where I wasn't able to have enough self-direction—one of my strongest motivators. I needed to have space for creative thinking and to implement innovative ideas. Some jobs just did not offer that opportunity. While I had been quite successful in my work over the years, I can see now that this was actually driven by my strong benevolence and universalism values, more so than the strength of my achievement values.

Also, after completing the activity, I had a much better idea about why my husband does certain things. I realised he has quite a different values profile compared to me. As someone who had been a serious athlete in his youth, achievement had been very strong in his values profile. I could see that this still drove him today in the things he focused on and accomplished. He was also more driven by personal security and had spent years focusing on the financial security of our family. Unlike me, he did not require a lot of stimulation in his employment and had been quite happy to stay in the same job for a number of years. His values, while they sometimes irritated and frustrated me, ensured there was in fact some balance in our household. His stability enabled me to be the one who tried to change the world. I, of course, knew none of this when we married, so it is a happy outcome that opposites do, in fact, attract!

All values are likely to have some influence over the issue of weight management, although some may have more impact than others. The following are examples of how particular value profiles may influence weight management.

People with strong achievement values

Such people would likely find weight management much easier than I do. Someone who valued success would be focused across a number of domains in their life. These may include success in the fields of business, study, academia, employment, sport, finances and, yes, weight management. These people would be naturally 'driven' and perhaps be described by others as 'focused' and 'hard working'. Achievers wouldn't mind spending hours and hours of their time aimed towards their success. They would be the ones who were likely to spend time training to improve their athletic skills or take on additional study to give themselves an edge at work. They could spend years working enormous hours to ensure a business venture succeeded. And they would also be the ones who looked at food as something that can increase or decrease their success. Therefore, their eating habits would be more rigid in nature.

People with strong personal security and conformity values

People with strong values here would have variable responses to weight management, depending on their circumstances. For example, someone who works in media, such as television, music, news or movies, is likely to be 'required' to maintain their weight at a certain level. It may be implied, or even enforced, that their careers would suffer if they did not maintain rigid control over their weight. These people would therefore demonstrate strong motivation due to the need to maintain their personal security through employment. Similarly, some people might find themselves in marriages or even social groups where the expectation is a certain level of weight management. Conforming and personal security are positioned close together on the wheel and so these things have a strong connection. People may feel socially insecure if they do not do things such as maintain an acceptable weight as endorsed by their social group.

People with strong face values

Someone with strong face values would be driven by an internal need to be viewed as attractive based on cultural social standards. Food and exercise would therefore be seen as a means to ensure this attractiveness is sustained and would be done with great self-discipline. Their motivation would come from a place of deep fear, though, because a break from this self-discipline would put their attractiveness in jeopardy. These people probably find it quite easy to manage their weight because food that is defined by them as 'bad' is likely to invoke a real sense of anxiety within them and would therefore be actively avoided. If they did indulge, they may be more likely to punish themselves with additional workouts or diet cleansings to address their fear of weight gain. While these people may maintain their weight, you do not want to be in this group. These people spend an enormous amount of time and energy on themselves and live with an endless anxiety—the anxiety of aging, normal body changes, self-maintenance and self-obsession. That is not something to be envied. The prettiest of them would never feel beautiful enough, every 'flaw' would be obsessed over, and every photo posed and photoshopped to perfection. It must be exhausting being in this group!

People with strong universalism-environment values

There is another group of people who may find weight management easier due to their strong values. The environmentalists or animal activists may have some strict eating regimes based on their ideals of sustainable eating or animal conservation. These people may also be more inclined to spend time in nature, participating in conservation activities or growing their own produce. They are not driven by looks or success, but by a set of ethical principles connected to their deeply set universalism values. The outcome though, may still be greater motivational ease with weight control.

If you have spent some time with body-obsessed people, you may have found that they can actually be quite dull. They constantly talk about what they eat (or often more to the point, what they don't eat). I know I have avoided asking some people to my house for dinner simply because I can't be bothered to think about all their dietary restrictions. If I invite someone to come to my house, I want to bake a cheesecake and have people actually eat it and enjoy it, not eat it with a sense of guilt and fear. After all, life is too short to live without cheesecake!

Our values profile is a logical and reasonable explanation for why we may struggle to motivate ourselves regarding weight management. They are deeply set, and consistent across our lifespan. They cannot be battled; if we try to battle, we will eventually lose.

So, at this point you may be wondering what your values profile actually looks like. There are online surveys you can work through that may help you gain some idea. The information I am providing here is based on Shalom Schwartz's work, so if you go down that path I would recommend looking for assessments based on his research. You might also be surprised that just observing what you are naturally 'drawn' to motivationally will give you considerable information. When time is tight or there is a conflict between things you need to do, ask yourself which choice is the one most consistently influencing your behaviour? You could also keep a diary and start to reflect on how your values 'pull' you in certain ways.

Avoiding conflict in values can be an important way to work with the values profile you have. For example, when I am very busy, I rarely exercise. In fact, every time I worked fulltime I gained weight. This is important information, as it lets me know that other things always win out motivationally when I am busy. As a result, part of my strategy to ensure I have the time and energy to take better care of myself has been to reduce my working hours to four days a week. The values conflict still exists, but, as a result of freeing up my time, it arises less often and I have more capacity to include exercise into my schedule.

Once you understand the concept that opposites exist within your values system, you can start to approach your motivation with more knowledge and stop getting frustrated with yourself for 'not prioritising exercise'. I have lost more emotional weight from this knowledge than from anything else in this book. Maybe that's the type of weight to focus on losing first!

CHAPTER 4

Hope for life in general

'Courage does not always roar. Sometimes courage is a quiet voice at the end of the day saying "I will try again tomorrow"'

— Mary Anne Radmacher

Hope is a profound driver of motivation. And a lack of hope can completely annihilate it. I have never seen anyone do anything with any degree of motivation without the presence of hope. As such, I have put it into the core motivational layers of the onion.

What's interesting to me is that I rarely hear hope linked strongly to the idea of motivation. The chapters on hope in this book, however, will be some of the most important you will read. The media describes our current state of health in Western society as an 'obesity epidemic'. That is true, but I believe that it is an epidemic largely being driven by hopelessness. In the next two chapters, I am going to discuss two differing types of hope:

1. General hope in life
2. Hope related to weight management.

I believe that many of the people we categorise as being obese will be experiencing one or both of these states of hopelessness.

What is hope?

Hope is a positive emotion based on the belief that things are possible. It is often a subconscious belief and therefore sits outside of people's awareness. Hope is the basis from which people are able to act or progress and, hence, is a strong driver of motivation. Psychologist and researcher C. R. Snyder studied hope and developed a theory about the components that enabled a person to have hope. He defined the components as follows:

1. Agency—a belief in personal capacity or ability
2. Pathways—seeing one or more ways to make progress.

Agency includes such things as believing we have the skills, knowledge, resources and energy to take on a challenge or activity. Pathways involve being able to recognise clear steps forward and seeing ways to manage challenges or barriers.

General hope in life

When I refer to general hope in life, I am referring to the idea that life, overall, is a positive experience. There is a sense of a future that can be looked forward to and will provide opportunity, fulfilment and joy. While there can be a recognition that struggles and suffering will occur, a person with general hope for life may believe they can manage the things that life throws at them.

I once asked a mental health client, 'When was the last time you felt hope?' He responded, 'I have never felt hope'. He was in his fifties and his whole experience of life had been one of hopelessness. Interestingly, this man was extremely obese, and there were teams of people trying to get him to lose weight. They were all failing miserably at this task, and after hearing him talk about hope, I knew why.

Hopelessness can be found in many places and within many people. Having worked in the field of mental health for twenty years, I have seen hopelessness at its most despairing and profound. I have seen people who are too hopeless to get out of bed, too hopeless to shower, too hopeless to speak. Some people grow up in an environment that sets them up for a life without hope, which is what had happened to my client. People with no hope don't act like people who care much about life. The lack of recognition about hopelessness is the key reason I struggled in the early part of my career. I was labelling it as a lack of motivation. Even if I had recognised this at the time, I wouldn't have had the skills or knowledge to work any differently. That has been a process that has taken me much longer.

I am now going to ask an important question. Do you have a life that is worth living? Do you actually live the type of life that you would happily live for many more years to come? Do you feel fulfilled, energised, happy and excited by your life? Or is your life a drudgery of habits and meaningless tasks? Are you stuck, disappointed or trapped in your life? I know it seems like a leap of judgement on my part, but if you are not living a life of authenticity and joy, it is likely to be having an impact on your motivation to manage your weight. Why? Because you are unlikely to be deeply driven to care for a life that is unfulfilling.

Keep in mind, this will be happening on a subconscious level. In essence, what I am saying is that, for us to genuinely and deliberately take care of our health, our wellbeing and, therefore, our life, we need to live a life that is worthwhile. Somewhere deep inside there may be a complacency about your health because your life isn't really what you want it to be.

Think of the client I mentioned above. He had *never* felt hope. I will reframe that for you. He had never lived a life where he felt he had a future worth fighting for. It was no accident that this man ended up obese. And it was no accident that he was not listening to the health advice about his weight. Why wouldn't he sacrifice his long-term health for a short-term sense of comfort through food? It is not logical to try and 'motivate' him to be healthy unless we first look at the underlying problem—a life worth living. It is absurd to ask people feeling this way to do more exercise and to watch what they eat.

Weight cannot be segregated into a biomedical issue. We can't just focus on calories in versus calories out. Human beings are not robots. They cannot be programmed to live by certain rules when it comes to exercise and eating. We are complex emotional and spiritual beings. And it is time to recognise this in how we support people with weight-related issues. As I said earlier, we can't just educate people into losing weight. We must understand the complex components that impact their ability to WANT to take care of their health.

My own story of hopelessness

I mentioned in the first chapter that there was a period in my life where I struggled with hopelessness. My son is now fifteen.

He is a funny, affectionate, engaging and an amazing human being. He also has autism and a significant developmental delay. While there are many moments of joy with him, the journey in raising him has also been challenging.

When I first came to the realisation that my child had a disability, I experienced an inevitable stage of grief and loss. The journey I expected to follow in raising my child was very different to the one I was now facing. But from the beginning, I had a sense that I had the capacity (or agency) to manage what this life would require. So, I had hope. There was also the worry that came with the journey—what do we do, how will his future look? Again, even though I didn't know the pathways available, I felt that there were options to be explored. And I therefore had hope. There was the exhaustion and the stress of day-to-day living, which at times was overwhelming. However, each time I sunk to a low point, I seemed to find the ability (agency) to pull myself up by the bootstrings and continue forward (pathways). And therefore, I had hope.

But one day, I really did lose hope.

Of course, it didn't happen in just one day, it happened over many years. But I did eventually lose the belief that I had the capacity (agency) and that I would find a way (pathways). And as a result, hope was gone. You see, there was one issue, despite my best efforts and the efforts of those around me, that had left me feeling completely and utterly powerless. My son was violent towards me every single day.

It was an issue that started slowly at first, with the occasional grabbing of my arms. We tried many things to manage it. We tried behavioural techniques where we gave him consequences; we tried reinforcement techniques, where we taught him acceptable behaviours; we tried calming techniques, where we gave him space; and in desperation we tried yelling and screaming techniques, which caused greater stress and more behavioural issues. We even tried medications at one point, which made things worse, not better. This went on for years and years. We went to experts, we looked at books, and we did things by trial and error. We found some things helped some of the time, but we couldn't seem to reduce the behaviours. In fact, as he was getting older, the behaviours were getting worse. And while he was hurting many people, including his father, teachers and babysitters, I was the one he targeted the most. He was scratching and pulling my hair every day, and I had to remain calm, loving and focused while I was being physically hurt. My beloved child was lashing out at me physically, and it truly felt hopeless.

His behaviour became so bad, we could barely leave the house. There were only a couple of locations where he felt safe enough and wouldn't have a meltdown. These places were the local supermarket and McDonald's. I couldn't take him on a plane to see grandparents, I couldn't take him to the park for a picnic, and I couldn't take him into a shopping centre to buy him shoes. Our house therefore became our life. Other than going to work, home was where we spent our time.

Any family activity couldn't be done as a family, unless it was done at home. Errands had to be done separately by my husband, Peter, and me, and activities for my daughter, Maya, had to be done with just one parent. We had no additional help other than the occasional visit from grandparents or the odd babysitter. It made us feel very alone in our problems. There was no magic wand—no program, no medicine, and no help.

So, we went into survival mode. We tried to make the best of it. We went swimming in our pool, we had barbecues, we baked cakes and we had pizza night. We gardened, we played with our dog and we looked at our beautiful ocean view. And we tried to have a semblance of a life that was joyful. But each day, the scratching and kicking and hair pulling continued. And the exhaustion and the despair escalated. We calmed him and soothed him and loved him through it all. But we stayed at home in our domestic prison and pretended we didn't need anything else to make us happy.

But the truth was, this wasn't a life worth living. My sole aim during this period was to get to the end of the day without completely losing it. It took every ounce of will to do so. I felt that I could survive the day, I could survive the week and I could survive the year. What I felt I couldn't survive was the next forty years of living this life. In the back of my mind was an image of myself at eighty being beaten by my now strong, adult son. While not suicidal, I did not have a strong attachment to the idea of a long life. I didn't want to kill myself, but I didn't want to take care of myself either. The idea of having a heart attack in my sixties was almost soothing. It would reduce the amount of time I had to cope.

One of my joys during this time was cooking. I could cook at home and I could do it while caring for my son. And so, every day I got up and cooked. I nailed an amazing cheesecake, I perfected a pavlova, and I created sticky date puddings, brownies, apple crumbles and lime tarts. I experimented with slow-cooked casseroles, soups and stews, roasts and grills, paellas and risottos. And I ate it, usually with a glass or two of fabulous wine. And I survived one day at a time. Because I cooked and I ate.

I knew I was not taking care of my health. I had given up on my health. I didn't care enough about my future life to care enough about my current health. And in a life that felt pretty joyless for a time, cooking and eating was one of the few joys I had available. And so, I gained weight. It was a necessary part of my survival. When I looked in the mirror I saw a woman who was chubby, but also a woman who was strong, determined and courageous—a survivor. I was not unmotivated, I was not lazy and I didn't have poor priorities. I took something joyful and held onto it for dear life. The fact that it made me fat doesn't take away from the fact that it also helped me survive through this period. It was rational and logical to do so at the time.

But I knew I was feeling hopeless and that this was driving my weight gain. I could therefore see it as a symptom of an overwhelming life. Just like the messy house, unironed clothes and disorganised cupboards. They were not the highest priorities at the time. As a result, I was able to have compassion for myself. This gave me a perspective that enabled me to see the weight for what it was—a sign of a really tough time.

Overall, this period probably lasted about three years. Eventually a pathway of hope developed that I could not have anticipated at the time. My son grew up and grew out of many of these behaviours. Again, it happened slowly. Somehow, he learnt to manage the negative feelings and anxieties better, and we slowly started to reintroduce outings and family activities into our lives again. The other hope-supporting factor came about because of a change in government policy in Australia: the National Disability Insurance Scheme was introduced. For the first time in my son's life we were actually able to access some help through this new funding model, which focused on the individual needs of people with a disability. This meant I could start to believe in a future where I wasn't eighty years old and still caring for my son.

The thing about hope, though, is that it takes courage and it takes proof. Hope returns cautiously—it comes and goes in waves. The more time that went by without troubling behaviours, the more I started to trust the feeling of hope again. But it only took one bad day for it to go crumbling backwards again. It only took one shred of doubt for me to think this could all be lost. Hope can't be conjured, it is an internal process that requires proof that things actually are getting better, and also the time to believe it. Even then, there is a doubt in the back of the mind that takes time and courage to heal. It is not a quick or easy process. So, I have been allowing myself the time to re-emerge into hope, without pressure, frustration or guilt.

Let's take a moment to think about what it would have been like for me if a well-meaning health professional brought up the issue of my weight in the midst of this hopelessness. What would my reaction have been, do you think? Would I have welcomed their concern and their advice? I think you can see the terrible timing for such a conversation, and it would have added to my sense of hopelessness. It would have made me feel even more alone in my problems. It would have frustrated and angered me. And yet I know that this is the type of thing happening every single day in the world of health. And it makes the problem worse, not better.

During this time of hopelessness, I was watching morning television when yet another segment aired about the obesity epidemic. The program had brought on a young, fit personal trainer to tell us 'some simple ways to lose weight'. She had the fashionable exercise gear on, showing her tiny waist and abs, her hair was in a pony tail that swung with enthusiasm from side to side, and she talked about how easy it was to do some squats and lunges in our living rooms. I picked up a cushion and threw it with fury at the television, saying something along the lines of 'You fucking bitch! Come and live my life for a couple of months!' The last person on the planet I needed telling me to get fit was someone like that. I probably bought a couple of donuts that day and perhaps had a bowl of ice-cream as well. All that story did was add to my sense of hopelessness.

Hope relates to motivation in all aspects of life, not just weight management. Lack of hope leads to people giving up on their marriages. Lack of hope leads to drug problems, crime and violence. Lack of hope leads to staying in jobs that are mediocre and dull. Lack of hope means not taking medications and not following doctor's instructions. Lack of hope means saying, 'This is the hand I've been dealt and I just need to accept it'. Lack of hope is actually protective. That is why we need to be very careful when people have lost hope in their lives. Psychologically, they are in a state of self-protection. That is not something that can be easily pulled down, and in fact needs to be managed very delicately. I have seen overzealous helpers come into the life of people who lack hope, only to find a very large wall facing them. In mental health, we would have called this a 'lack of engagement'. People with low hope will not let you into their lives easily. They will test you over many months before they let you anywhere near their real thoughts and feelings. People who try and sledgehammer through the protective wall with their enthusiasm will find themselves shunned extremely quickly. And frankly, this is an important act of self-protection.

Finding hope out of hopelessness is an incredibly courageous move. It opens that person up to things they are terrified of, things they have often already experienced, things they have failed at, and things that they feel could destroy them once and for all. Think of a puppy that has experienced abuse. It is a long road for the puppy to experience trust. Human beings in a state of hopelessness are exactly the same. Time and a lot of evidence are required to even begin to move into a state of hopefulness again.

If you currently feel that hopelessness for life in general is an issue you are facing, worrying about weight loss is probably not the place to start. Hope for life in general requires a much broader focus and now might not be the time to try and change it. It may in fact take some help from someone qualified and experienced in working with people in states of hopelessness. This will depend on how deeply embedded the state of hopelessness feels to you. If you think it is just about boredom and reinvigorating your life, it may just be introducing some new goals to energise your life. If it feels all-encompassing, however, you may want to seek out some professional help.

While hope for life in general and motivation for weight loss may seem unrelated, they are in fact much more closely related than you think. Kindness towards yourself and a recognition of the impact of hope on your life and overall wellbeing is a starting place to accepting what seems like a 'lack of motivation' when it comes to your weight.

CHAPTER 5

Hope for weight management

'When you're at the end of your rope, tie a knot and hold on'

— Theodore Roosevelt

It would be rare to find an overweight person who hasn't tried to lose weight. In fact, most people would have made a number of genuine attempts. And many of these attempts would have been successful or at least partially successful—for some time at least. Let's face it, exercise and calorie restriction does result in weight loss. The problem though is that, in the vast majority of cases, the motivational capacity of people to sustain these behaviours over time is limited. And inevitably, that leads to a regain of the weight.

Let's think about the impact of this process on hope. Imagine you are trying to lose weight. To even attempt to lose weight, you would need hope that weight loss was possible. Hope would have come in the form of a new diet plan, a paid program or a current fad. Inevitably, you would have seen people who had been 'successful' in this new strategy and you would launch yourself into it with commitment, and inevitably experience a little bit of success. This would feel nice and people would start to comment. All the things people told you do in fact work—exercise with a friend, plan your meals, set a goal, don't keep temptation in your fridge and stick to a routine. It could even feel easy for a while! You may wonder why you didn't try this earlier.

Eventually people would start to really notice a difference and ask you what you were doing to achieve such success. You would be delighted to tell them about your new program. Once you get to the point where your clothes are loose, you might be brave enough to go and purchase some new clothes. It would be exciting to realise you are a size smaller, and you'd get a little buzz as you make your new purchases. Eventually you get brave enough to post something on social media, perhaps even in your exercise gear! You get a flurry of encouragement that drives you on with even greater enthusiasm.

Then you hit your goal weight. Hooray! You are flushed with your success. You can't imagine going back to your old ways! You talk about how much energy you have with anyone who will listen, you munch on your salads, and you avoid alcohol and dessert. You feel great! And you look great too—everyone says so! And this can go on for a while, sometimes even for a year or two.

And then something happens.

You gain a little bit of weight. Not much at first, but enough to get you 'focused again'. So, you do some extra workouts and are very careful with your food intake. Some of the weight comes off, but there seems to be a 'few stubborn kilos' you can't quite shift this time. You're not happy about it, but you don't let it get you down. You stick to your routines, only occasionally treating yourself or missing an exercise session. You manage to keep the weight at bay for a while longer. But then you have a bout of sickness or an injury that throws out your fitness routine. On top of that you've had an extra busy time at work and have needed to stay back late. Your child also gets into the state soccer trials and needs to attend extra training sessions, putting additional pressure on the family routine. This is all topped off by a holiday in which the cocktails were half price during happy hour, and you felt it only right to enjoy them! You tentatively get on the scales and are horrified by what you see. How could you have gained so much weight again? Hope starts to wane, but you are not prepared to give into it.

Depressed, you punish yourself. You exercise to the point of exhaustion and starve yourself for a couple of weeks. Again, the weight starts to come off. But a bad week at work leaves you sobbing over a bowl of pasta carbonara followed by a chocolate brownie. You've really blown it now, so you go for a second brownie and seriously consider a third. You feel pathetic and berate yourself for having no willpower. Hopelessness really starts to take over. Your partner comments on the change in your routine and may even mention the extra weight. You show them who the boss is by throwing back a couple of glasses of wine and half a block of brie.

The fat pants you had hidden at the back of the cupboard come out again. Your buttoned shirts start to bulge. Every Monday becomes the start of your new diet, only to be given up by

Wednesday. Hope feels a long way off now. You can't remember how you were managing to do it before. Workout sessions occur less and less often, and, before you know it, you are back to your old weight. Deeply depressed, you no longer attempt to manage your weight. Why bother? You are exhausted from the effort and it didn't work anyway. You throw in the towel and decide you are going to be fat and happy. For a while you embrace it, convincing yourself you really do love it. You eat pizza with extra cheese and don't see any big deal in eating chocolate croissants for breakfast every day—the French do it after all! Until you weigh yourself again or go up yet another clothing size. And then you feel like a complete failure. What is wrong with you?

There is a very clear answer to that question: absolutely nothing. If this story has any degree of familiarity to you, it is because you have acted like a completely normal, rational human being! You have not demonstrated your deficiencies or your flaws—you have demonstrated your normalcy. Congratulations, you are not a screw-up!

Let's go back to how the story emerged. It starts with a feeling of hope in which you believed you had the ability (agency) and a plan (pathway) that would finally work for you. You would have been convinced that this new pathway would work because it is better than the last pathway you took to try and lose weight. You saw the success stories after all, and they had a very detailed explanation as to why this plan would work when others didn't. There may have even been some complicated scientific evidence thrown at you that sounded extremely convincing. They would have used the term 'clinical trials' just to add weight to the argument.

But let me tell you something about diets and weight management. In my opinion, the same people who were thin when we all did the low-fat diets are the very same people who are now thin using the Paleo or low-carb diets. It is NOT the diet or eating plan that is enabling them to be thin, it is their motivational profile. They are driven to be thin because of their deep motivational nature. They are not thin because they cut out carbs. It is their level of conscious focus on food and exercise, which is driven by their motivational natures, that is the cause of their success with weight management.

If you struggle to be thin, you will struggle to be thin no matter what diet plan you adopt. By trying to use the same techniques and strategies that people who are strongly motivated for weight management use, you will place yourself in a very dangerous category—a weight cycler category. That is the worst category to be in—both physically and motivationally. Weight cyclers go up and down with their weight, time and time again, over many years. They are NOT healthy and they are NOT thin (at least not consistently). They also end up feeling hopeless about managing their weight.

People who weight cycle go through extremes. They go from strong hope (when they take on a diet) to deep hopelessness (when they are unable motivationally to sustain the diet). They do extreme things to their bodies when they feel hope, and they then do extreme things to their bodies when they feel hopeless. They will ban any 'bad food' (as defined by the new diet plan) and follow this with zealous enthusiasm, and they will then eat with complete abandon and disregard for their health when the latest diet has failed (due to their sense of hopelessness). It is the extremes that create the problem and the reason why people who diet in long-term studies are fatter than people who never diet. The people who never diet avoid this motivational pattern of extremes. And it is much better for them physically and motivationally to do so. I am not against diets because they do not help us lose weight, I am against diets because they have a long-term impact on hope that is far more dangerous to our health. They give us false hope, and false hope is a direct pathway to hopelessness. This is motivationally normal. We don't 'fail' at diets—diets fail full stop.

The majority of the sixty per cent of Australians who are currently overweight have dieted at some point in their life. And yet they are still overweight. It's time we stopped blaming people for this failure and started blaming the strategies we've used. Failing at diets is normal human behaviour. It is predictable human behaviour. Einstein's definition of insanity was to keep using the same technique and expecting a different outcome. And yet how many people do you know who are currently 'on a diet'. How many times have you tried this strategy yourself? Diets predicably fail, and I would also say, predictably lead to hopelessness. And hopelessness leads to giving up small, health related behaviours that are in fact making a difference.

The pattern of hopelessness causes people to completely give in. When we focus solely on the number on the scales and keep telling people they are overweight, we drive them in the direction of diets. But diets don't work, and diets cause damage. The thing that is most important in managing weight and health in the longer term is all the little things we are doing day to day that stop the problem from getting worse. Hopelessness leads to an abandonment of all these little things. We go from an occasional soft drink as a treat, to guzzling it like water. We go from one scoop of ice-cream to two. We go from a twenty-minute walk once a week to none at all. We throw in the towel. And this is the most dangerous scenario we can be in as a society—because now we have thousands if not millions of people who have thrown in the towel on weight management. When we focus just on what the scale says, we fail to recognise the critical role of these small behaviours. People, in their continuous effort to keep losing weight, are giving up their best defence for long-term health outcomes—stopping or minimising further weight gain. No one needs three brownies, but hopelessness leads people to a place that makes this seem reasonable.

I currently work in a job where I sit between seven to eight hours a day. If I am not at my computer, I am in meetings. The only activity I get during a workday is walking to and from these meetings and the occasional walk-around the hospital to talk to patients or staff. I do schedule meetings and volunteer to go to another person's office just to try and get a few more 'steps' into my day.

When I get home from work, I usually go straight about preparing dinner. My son's disability requires a considerable amount of hands-on caring, so we are still required to help him toilet, bathe, dress, brush his teeth and prepare for bed. There is also the washing-up, not to mention the laundry that needs to be done. Throw in there, somewhere, helping my daughter with homework, checking emails, paying bills or filling in school permission notes, and before you know it the evening is almost over. At some point I crash and manage to watch an hour of TV before crawling into bed for an exhausted sleep.

While I mostly cook fresh meals, inevitably we eat one or two pre-prepared meals a week, and at least one take-away. In the rush to get to work in the mornings, I don't always have time to prepare a lunch. There are plenty of options to purchase at work, which I will take advantage of on those days.

Weekends are a jam of activities and chores. Grocery shopping, kids' sleepovers, art classes, swimming lessons, cleaning, laundry, gardening and errands. If I see a friend at all on a weekend, it feels like a luxury. My life is an average modern Western life. Despite this, I manage to walk the dog a few times a week, do a couple of fifteen-minute yoga sessions and perhaps swim once or twice in the hot season. I think I am actually doing pretty well to manage this much!

Let's add on top of this all the messages we have about being healthy. Apparently, we're supposed to be eating five serves of vegetables a day, although ninety-five per cent of Australians are not doing this at present. We keep hearing statistics that tell us we are overweight and obese, and how fat our children are. We are bombarded with thin fitness images, ponytails swinging, telling us that it is easy and we just need 'better priorities'. On top of that, television shows, movies, magazines, advertisements and pretty much anything else show us young, thin, fit people. We then go to the GP to be told we are ten kilos overweight and really need to 'find some motivation'. Our friend posts an image on Facebook after having lost weight on some new magic pill that only costs $200 a month. Our child comes home from school and tells us the sausages we are cooking for dinner (because that's all that was left in the freezer) are in fact bad for us, which they learnt today in their school health program. We go to our favourite clothing store to buy something nice, only to realise we are now too fat to wear anything they have in stock, and are relegated, quite quickly, into dowdy fashion. A letter arrives home from preschool reminding us that the muffin we packed is on the 'banned foods' list, and please don't do it again. We only did it because all we could find was a bruised and rotten apple at the bottom of the fridge, and we know a fed kid is better than hungry kid. We hoped, somehow, we'd get away with it. We didn't.

So, what do we do? Crack open a chocolate and sit on the couch to binge-watch *Orange is the New Black*. Why? Because we've been trying. And we are failing—miserably. Are we really surprised by the fact that people are feeling hopeless about managing their weight? We do care about our health, but unless we feel we have agency and pathways when it comes to our weight, we'll just give ourselves a break and pick up takeaway for dinner.

So, what can be done? Are we all doomed to morbid obesity? No, I don't believe we are. But we must protect our hope from these messages that continually tell us we are not doing well enough no matter how hard we try. Have you ever actually tracked just how much you manage to do in a day? Have you ever listed all the things you do that help with your health? I can guarantee you are doing far more than you think. And *this* is the place to start when it comes to hope for weight management—recognising the fact that you do have knowledge, skills and abilities when it comes to weight management (or as Snyder called it, agency). Diets take you to extremes of hope, and the environment is adding another barrage of hopelessness to the equation. The inundation of health information is overwhelming and makes us feel like failures. For most of us, we feel this daily, which is not a recipe for hope.

Hope is in and of itself a very complex issue. Rebuilding hope for weight management is something that takes time and requires skilled support. I have found that a little bit of information can be dangerous in the wrong hands, which makes me somewhat reluctant to give information that may be misconstrued and used by people with no skill or knowledge in complex psychological phenomena. Even skilled and experienced therapists don't always understand the sophistication of hope. As such, I will say this: the aim of this book and this information is to support your hope. Through the process of realising the problem is not a deficit within you, I aim to help you take a step towards hopefulness when it comes to your weight—not hope to be skinny but hope to be healthy. Hope to feel good about yourself and the body you have. Hope to create a new world that understands the complexity of motivation. This book is just the start of a bigger picture towards hopefulness when it comes to weight management.

CHAPTER 6

Passion

---

*'Above all be true to yourself.
And if you cannot put your heart into it,
take yourself out of it.'*

— Hardy D. Jackson

There are some things in life we just love doing. Some people collect dolls, others immerse themselves in books, some are obsessed with the weather, and there are those who spend hours watching birds. There is no explanation as to why we as individuals are drawn to certain interests. We often look at each other's interests and shake our heads, wondering why someone would even want 4,000 pieces of Elvis Presley memorabilia, but hey, each to their own.

A passion is an interest so strong that we start to identify ourselves by it. Someone who likes painting might say, 'I paint', but someone who is passionate about it would say, 'I am a painter'. It is a subtle difference, but it indicates the depth of commitment (or motivation) that the person has for the activity. I am a writer. It took me a long time to say that though, because it felt a bit pretentious. I wasn't always a writer, which is why I think it took me a long time to adjust to calling myself one. I didn't start to write until I was in my late thirties and I had something I felt I needed to write about. Now though, after a few years, I am happy to say it is not only a passion of mine, but my true purpose and nature to write.

I also have a passion for food. Again, I would struggle to call myself a 'foodie' because television shows have made that look elitist. But I don't have a 'bucket list', I have a 'food and beverage bucket list'. These are the some of the things that are on that list:

- Drink a bottle of wine that costs more than $100.
- Take a cooking class in Italy.
- Learn to make awesome pork crackling.
- Grow a lemon and lime tree.
- Meet Jamie Oliver (because you have to dream big).
- Make a croquembouche.
- Eat escargot in France.

I am more inclined to buy beautiful serving platters than I am shoes (although shoes are good too). You may have guessed from my bucket list that my favourite celebrity chef is Jamie Oliver. I was incredibly impressed after watching him do his series where he aimed to change the quality of food served in British schools. There's a man who understands what we need to be doing when it comes to obesity in our communities! My ultimate Jamie Oliver fantasy would be to have him come to my house and cook. I could sit at the kitchen bench and watch him while sipping a glass of crisp white wine. We would talk food and he would use fancy cooking words like *beurre blanc* before whipping out his latest Jamie Oliver custom designed zester. I would show him my herb garden, and he'd be impressed by the size of the chillies, before grabbing a handful of fresh dill to add to the meal. We'd eat his amazing food and barely talk in order to savour each mouthful. There would be more wine and laughter before passing out in a food coma on the lounge! Bliss!

As mentioned earlier, I also like to cook. I will put on my apron and conjure my 'inner Jamie' while chopping and stirring and tasting—all with a glass of wine in hand. I am a reasonable cook, although nothing like those people you see in cooking competitions on television. I only like to cook under specific circumstances—when I have enough time and feel relaxed. This means weeknight cooking is not something I particularly enjoy. Under these circumstances I am like any other busy mother or father in the kitchen, cooking the quickest and easiest dish I can find, while trying to get my kids to eat a reasonable meal!

Dinner with children is one of the most stressful parts of parenting. My poor colleagues have endured years of my debriefing about children and their eating (or lack of it). I have apparently helped them though, as they have gone on to have their own children and their own food battles. They now know this is normal behaviour for children! I have no tips except for perseverance. It does eventually get better, although much slower than any of us would like! My mother put this into perspective for me one day. She grew up in a poor home and told me that each day they ate exactly the same thing—wheat biscuits for breakfast, jam sandwiches for lunch and post-school snacks (on white bread), and meat with two vegetables (always potatoes and either carrots or peas) for dinner. They would occasionally have dessert, which was a cake or tart with custard. Fruit was expensive and saved for her father to take to work. My mother says she didn't eat a salad until she was twenty-one! This story soothed me as a young mother struggling with food guidelines and the pressure of raising healthy children. My mother has been a very healthy person, so it's something to keep in mind.

As far as I am concerned, food is one of the great joys in life and it should be enjoyed fully and wholeheartedly. For me, it is an essential part of a life well lived—a life of love and music and dance and travel and sex and laughter. The thought of eating only for health has much appeal to me as having sex only to conceive children. You can educate me until the cows come home, but I am still going to eat cheesecake.

I had a foodie friend called Kym who lived up the road for about a year. I'd send her a text message that would simply say 'Paella?' And she'd respond with 'I'll bring the wine'. Or 'Osso bucco?' and she'd say, 'I've got a camembert in the fridge'. The routine was that she'd sit at the kitchen bench and chat while I cooked. We would have a glass of wine and a good cheese while the cooking was happening. She'd set the table and took over the dishes after dinner. While we ate, there was always a discussion such as, 'Do you think there's enough chilli in this?', and she'd say, 'Yes, but it would probably be even better with a bit more'. Or I'd ask, 'Can you taste the lemon zest I added?' And she'd proclaim, 'I wondered what that was!' There's something about having someone who really appreciates food when you cook and is happy to discuss the ingredients in detail. My husband loves my cooking, but if I ask a question the answer is always, 'It tastes great to me'. I once spent hours making a bolognaise sauce. I tended to it over those hours, constantly tasting and adding things as I went. I was trying to get the right balance between the tomato flavours and the beef stock. It had home grown herbs in it, and I added a touch of lemon zest just before I finished—a tip I learnt from Jamie to 'add a fresh twist to a rich dish'. Bless you, Jamie! I had the first bite and thought, 'Oh my god, this is the best bolognaise I've ever made!' I said to my family, 'What do you think?' My husband said, 'It's okay'. My son had one mouthful and wouldn't eat anymore. And my daughter said, 'Yeah, it's pretty good'. I really missed Kym that day—she would have noticed the lemon zest! When she moved from our street she went to live in Perth, on the other side of the country. She was so excited about a bottle of wine from a local vineyard, she sent me one in the post. The postage would have cost her more than the wine! That's a true foodie friend! It was awesome by the way, and I rang her to talk about it while I sipped a glass.

One of the things I find interesting is that the cultures that enjoy food like I do are also the cultures that are healthier. Research conducted twenty years ago showed that people who perceived food as a means of pleasure more so than health were ironically the ones who had better health outcomes. Why was this? Had we turned food into something to be anxious about? Did every mouthful induce guilt and fear, or a sense of deprivation? Having watched my colleagues eat lunch for twenty years, it seems perhaps this was the case. There was always a discussion such as 'I'm being bad today' or 'I'm trying to be good'. I think people who really enjoy food are also more likely to take the time to find good ingredients and are more likely to be mindful of their food, eating each mouthful with joy. I will always be passionate about food. There is no explanation as to why I am like this—it is just a part of who I am.

Let's talk about other people's passions though. My husband is passionate about fitness. When I first met him, he was competing in triathlons but he also had a history of competing in athletics. As a teenager, he was a long-jumper and 100-metre sprinter, and he was very talented at both—so much so that he spent his teenage years training with the aim of going to the Olympics. Unfortunately, an ongoing injury interrupted this dream, but he never lost his passion for fitness and training.

Years ago, we had a Category 5 cyclone (hurricane) called Yasi bear down upon our tropical city of Townsville. Thankfully, we didn't get a direct hit from the eye of the storm, but it was still quite scary. In typical fashion, my husband was out jogging the morning Yasi was due to arrive! Everyone else was in a panic, preparing their homes, but he needed to go out and run. After the storm had passed the city was covered in fallen trees and branches, so much so that you couldn't drive on the roads. What did my husband do? Went out for another run. When I suggested that it might be dangerous to run through storm debris, he shrugged off my concerns. Even when he has been sick, I have had conversations suggesting that training was not the most sensible thing for him to be doing. He has to be really sick to agree with me though! I can't fight this passion in him, no matter how logical my argument. It is a deep, intrinsic need he has to exercise. I know he will be that eighty-year-old who is still lifting weights in the nursing home—probably while hanging onto his walker!

Sometimes I find this intrinsic motivation for exercise annoying—why can't he be like a 'normal' person and sleep in occasionally? But, of course, the answer is that this is his 'normal'. It is not mine however, and no matter how hard I try, it never will be. I have tried to get up at five am to exercise like he does. It lasts about two days. I like to exercise, but I am not an 'exerciser'. If I am too busy or overwhelmed, or if the weather isn't right, I will not be motivated to exercise. My husband however will exercise under any circumstances—including when cyclones are nearby! That is the difference between people who are passionate about something and people who just like something. The motivational drive sits in a completely different space. He has a strong motivational drive to exercise and I have a weak one. Having a passion for fitness and exercise is quite handy in this day and age. It means the likelihood of being obese is greatly reduced. But this passion is obviously something only some people have, and it is not a choice.

The reality is that many of the people who work in the fitness industry have the same passion as my husband. They are probably the ones who were great at sport as children and spent all their time training and attending sporting events. Fitness to them feels natural, motivating and interesting. In fact, they may become anxious when they don't exercise and feel 'wrong' somehow. And they end up choosing professions related to their passion. My husband's original intent when he became a psychologist was to be a sports psychologist. Walk into any hospital and you can immediately pick the physiotherapists (physical therapists)—they are the ones who look like they spend their weekends rowing and cycling. Physical education teachers, exercise physiologists and personal trainers all will have had an interest in sport and fitness from a young age. This is no accident of course!

But what happens when you have a group of professionals who all have a really strong passion for sport and fitness (and therefore really strong motivational drivers) working with a group of people who do not? The group of people they are working with usually have a different motivational profile and the fitness professionals do not comprehend the people who are not strongly motivated by sport and exercise. And vice versa. What then happens is you have a group of professionals who are passionate about fitness trying to convince these other people to 'get motivated'. They tend to use the same thinking that works for them because that is what they know. These are the get up at five am people. They cannot understand the 'I'd rather stay in bed thank you' people they are trying to help. As a result, they tend to see it as a simple choice and a matter of priorities, because that is what it *feels* like to *them*. Unfortunately, it is just not that simple.

Let me give you an example of what this is like for those of us without a passion for fitness and sport. Did you know that knitting is also a health-enhancing activity? It is relaxing and requires considerable cognitive skill, which leads to a healthy brain and all the benefits of relaxation to the body. What if doctors and the government decided to try and motivate everyone to knit because of its health-enhancing benefits? Suddenly we would see an influx of knitting groups. We'd see messaging in doctors' waiting rooms and on television about the benefits of knitting. Research would start to look more closely at what type of knitting worked best, and how often people needed to knit to gain the most benefit. People at work would talk about the need to knit and how they are trying to work it into their busy schedules. We may have knitting competitions between colleagues to see who could do the most stitches in a day! Marketers would catch on and there'd be all sorts of new knitting paraphernalia such as special knitting chairs, knitting lights and knitting books. They might even invent knitting outfits! The knitters would love this and would celebrate their success at being healthy. They'd even wear their knitting outfits to the coffee shop with pride.

Knitters might start to brag about it and post their latest knitting accomplishments on social media. They would get plenty of 'likes' and comments such as 'keep up the good work' or 'I can't believe your motivation'. People might get knitting envy. They could look at these posts and feel like failures. Why can't I get motivated to knit like they do? The knitters would tell them you've just got to set a schedule and stick to it. Get up at five am to do your knitting before you go to work. Or start a knitting group and knit with other people! There'd be an influx of knitting blogs and knitting memes with inspirational quotes. They'd encourage you to give yourself a reward when you've completed your knitting goal! Then you just need to maintain your knitting habit for the rest of your life! Easy, right? Just set the goal and stick to it. No excuses please!

But if you're not a knitter, you're not a knitter. A person who is a runner is not going to suddenly become a knitter just because they've been 'educated' about the benefits. They can't just become a knitter because they set a goal. And they certainly don't want to get up at five am to knit so they can fit it into their busy schedule. It is absurd to think everyone would embrace knitting, just as it is absurd to expect everyone to embrace fitness.

But that is what the fitness message feels like to people who don't have a passion for it. I am neither a knitter nor a runner.

I do not want to get up at five am for either of these activities. I am therefore 'unmotivated'. And there are millions of other people in the world just like me. I can't change this and neither can they. Everyone with a passion for fitness needs to understand they have *different motivational drivers*. We are different from you. And pray that knitting doesn't become the new health fad! Can you imagine your doctor suddenly telling you that it is essential to knit at least three times a week, whether you like it or not?

And for all those people out there who are passionate knitters—good job. You are doing something positive for your health, so keep up the good work! But I won't be joining your knitting group, under any circumstances.

CHAPTER 7

Autonomy

'Because to take away a man's freedom of choice, even his freedom to make the wrong choice, is to manipulate him as though he were a puppet and not a person.'

— Madeleine L'Engle

Most people hate being told what to do. I would say it traumatises me. That may sound like a complete overreaction, and perhaps it is. But nonetheless, it is my reality. We all have a deep need to be autonomous and this seems to be a part of our human nature. Intrinsic motivation decreases when extrinsic motivation is applied as a means of trying to protect our autonomy from manipulation or coercion. This happens even when it goes against our best interests!

There are some people in the world who have had their autonomy threatened more than others. Not done with poor intention, this can occur when people find themselves on the receiving end of excessive or unsolicited advice. If you ask a parent of a child with a disability, they will tell you about being bombarded with other people's opinions. Ask any person who is obese and I believe you will hear exactly the same thing. As humans, we want to help. If we see what seems to be a reasonable or simple solution, we feel obligated to share it. The fact that this opinion may be based on a lack of understanding, or can come across as patronising, never seems to occur to us. But we have all felt that flash of anger and frustration that occurs when people overstep their boundaries and try to tell us how to live our lives.

What happens to people when this occurs over and over again, for many years, and from many different people or perspectives? What are the psychological consequences of threatened autonomy? In my life I would say it has been traumatic. It has led to a drive to protect myself from any further assaults on my autonomy. When you have a child with a disability you get more opinions and advice than you can imagine—from strangers, from doctors, from teachers, from television shows, from therapists, from families and from friends. I was at the local aquarium one day with my son, who was eating a sandwich, when a complete stranger came up and asked with outrage, 'You don't give him gluten do you?' In her opinion, gluten was causing all my son's problems. I had a waitress at a restaurant say to me, 'You know people with autism are really smart. You should focus on his strengths.' I had a substitute teacher ask me, 'Have you ever considered taking him to speech therapy?' after years of doing just that. I had an optometrist shame me for removing my son from therapy programs (to give us all a break) by telling me, 'You should know better'. I have had family members question why I wasn't taking him from doctor to doctor, and ask, 'Do you think steroids would help with his muscle strength?' I have had doctors tell me he must go to a special education school, and others who have told me he must not. I have had colleagues tell me that they would abort a baby if they knew it had a disability, but clarify, 'Of course, you wouldn't have known that in your case'. I have had a participant in a workshop tell me that 'disabled people should be put back into institutions where they can be taught how to behave properly rather than living with their rich parents and personal carers'. I have heard politicians say that children with autism stop other children from learning and should be separated from the ones who actually have some 'potential to contribute to society'. And I am not in any way unusual as the parent of a child with disability.

Opinions may seem benign, but they are not. They are exhausting. And at some point, you find yourself avoiding as many people as possible, just to escape the opinions—even when that includes the people you love. The only way to survive is to build a wall, and the more people that are involved, the stronger and taller the wall needs to be. What that looks like to other people is irrational or oversensitive behaviour. But when it comes to opinions, there is a cumulative impact. They become one whole overwhelming and exhausting force in life. And the pushback is equal to the whole, not the one small opinion people may have been expressing at the time.

This confuses people, as they perceive they are just trying to be helpful. But I, like many, am never fighting against one or two opinions, I'm fighting for my personal autonomy against hundreds of opinions. I have seen the same dynamic over and over again in my practice as a mental health practitioner. People seem to lose connection with 'common sense' and can even appear aggressive. Either that or resigned to be compliant—often both of these at different times.

Autonomy is a basic human need according to the researchers Ryan and Deci. They spent decades looking at how autonomy influenced motivation and determined it was a key component. What may seem unusual is that when people feel their autonomy is being threatened, they are actually inclined to do the exact opposite of what the person tells them to do. If you are obese, you probably know exactly what I am talking about. How many times have you been given advice about your weight and then left to go searching for a hamburger and fries? It is a normal assertion of your autonomy. Go to the bathroom at a Narcotics Anonymous meeting and I can guarantee you that someone is in there buying drugs just after leaving the meeting. Have a boss that is strict about leaving on time, and you will find a group of people sneaking out early when the boss isn't there. Tell a two-year-old they've watched enough Wiggles for the day, and all they want to do is watch more Wiggles.

Again, the thing to understand is that this behaviour is completely normal and, in fact, predictable. We all have an instinct to rebel when we feel we are being 'managed' by someone else. I always think our adult relationships with our parents are a good example of this autonomy need. Our parents believe they are giving us some sage advice, but adult children often have no time for it, whether the advice is good or not! What tends to happen is that we create an alternative argument in our minds *against* the advice we are being given. We start to discredit the information and come up with as many explanations as we can as to why the advice is wrong.

Let's consider something outside of the weight issue to demonstrate this dynamic. My friend's parents would like her to become a nurse. They speak to her about it often and give her all the reasons why being a nurse would be a great employment move: lots of career options, good money, steady employment, travel opportunities, etc. All these reasons are good and valid reasons. There is just one big problem. My friend does not want to be a nurse. She provides many explanations for not wanting to be a nurse, including the fact that she doesn't find it interesting. However, her parents don't believe her reasons outweigh the benefits they can clearly articulate. The discussion goes nowhere. The more they discuss the benefits, the more my friend believes the negatives, and the more she convinces herself *she just doesn't want to be a nurse.* Unwittingly, the parents are in fact reinforcing all the explanations as to why she doesn't want to be a nurse. Instead of being somewhat open-minded and objective about the idea, she is now completely and utterly biased towards never being a nurse. By impeding her autonomy to make her own decisions, her parents have in fact driven her towards the opposite argument. She is not thinking, 'Gee, my parents have a point'; instead, she is thinking, 'My parents are completely wrong' and will be able to list all the reasons in her mind as to why.

I'm pretty sure we can all recognise something like this in our own lives. As adults, we like to make our own choices and feel in charge. Having people tell us what to do causes us to immediately think of all the reasons against their argument or advice. We actually become biased towards the opposite argument as a result. This has been known for decades in the field of drug and alcohol counselling. The worst thing you can do is tell an alcoholic they must stop drinking. The problem arises because this information is not well known in most other areas of health or within the community. So, we have a lot of people using a technique that literally *drives people towards the opposite behaviour*. You can see where I am going here.

There's an advertisement on television at the moment that asks, 'What's your relationship with alcohol?' Every time I see it I want to pour myself a glass of wine. I have shown groups of people anti-smoking advertisements and asked them how they feel while watching them. The smokers in the group have all told me it makes them want to go and have a cigarette. This is even the case when the advertisement is meant to horrify and scare them by showing a smoker coughing up blood. It has the *opposite* impact than that intended. These are all examples of autonomy in action.

So, this creates a dilemma regarding how we manage the obesity epidemic, because the more we tell people what to do, the more likely they are to do the opposite. The more messages we receive, the stronger our autonomy drive will be. In my personal example, the pushback against advice was equal to the whole, not the single message or piece of advice. That is why I threw a cushion at energetic ponytail girl and her top fitness tips—the need to assert my autonomy.

A very wise therapist, Brian Cade, told me early in my career, 'Never be more motivated about the goal than your client'. He said this because he understood the basic human need to maintain autonomy. We have an internal radar that alerts us when someone is trying to get us to do something. The catch is that sometimes you don't even have to say anything to trigger the response. In my experience, people can sense the energy of someone else wanting them to coerce them. My friend's parents wouldn't even have to mentioned nursing now—any discussion about careers would be enough to cause tension. Her parents may see her as 'oversensitive' and 'irrational' on the issue, and on some level they are right. But they created the autonomy reaction that directly led to this result. So now we have a scenario where my friend says, 'My parents are pushy and won't listen', and her parents say, 'She just won't listen to common sense'. All it has achieved is frustration on both sides!

I have seen people trying to pretend they don't want to impede another person's autonomy, but if it is their intention to manipulate, the person will still know. You can't hide a desire to get someone else to change. Here's another clincher: I have also seen people's *enthusiasm* trigger someone's autonomy response. People can be so happy and excited for you that they in fact start to own the goal with you. I see this a lot with young therapists. Keen to help, they are just so excited to be out in the world working and helping people, and they fail to recognise that their enthusiasm for helping can sometimes come across as a bit *pushy*. Remember, never be more enthusiastic about the goal than the client! Some of the wisest words I have ever heard. For years, I deliberately had this statement written above my desk and, if I was struggling to engage with a client, I would ask myself, 'Am I more enthusiastic about this than they are?' The answer was often yes. I *really, really* wanted them to get a job because I thought it would make their life so much better. Or I *really, really* wanted them to stop smoking marijuana and improve their wellbeing. Or I *really, really* wanted them to do some exercise and lose some weight so they would have more energy. What happened though? They generally started avoiding me, which we would have labelled in their medical notes as a 'lack of engagement'. My enthusiasm was impeding their autonomy.

As a team leader of a mental health team, we once had a referral come through for which I said to the clinician who would be managing the client's case, 'Do not set a goal with this man for at least a year'. She looked at me dumbfounded and asked, 'What am I supposed to do with him then?' I told her, 'Your one aim is to gain his trust and let him know we don't want to control his life'. When I had seen his history, this man had spent decades in care with mental health services and had even had a number of stints in jail. His entire adult life would have felt controlled and managed. I knew we would get nowhere unless we gave him some space and let him know that he was safe to make his own decisions. After all that time, he would have been completely overreactive to another person with another plan and another set of goals. Interestingly, after six months he actually started to talk to us rather than just grunt during his appointments. After twelve months, he was setting his own goals and making his own plans without any interference or 'encouragement' from us. We had demonstrated to him that we weren't there to run his life, and as a result he was making progress. Any helper has an overwhelming need to help. But sometimes that gets in the way of what can actually be helpful.

Now of course, advice and encouragement doesn't need to come in the form of a person sitting across from us. Often it comes from advertisements, health campaigns and culture. The autonomy dynamic still exists with this type of advice though. We can get just as cranky at a television commercial as we can at a doctor or a spouse telling us what to do! As I've said before, we are barraged with information and expectations from our culture about weight. I believe the combined effect triggers an autonomy instinct in many of us. It's not just the one message that we hear occasionally, it is a constant and overwhelming stream of them. They might all be saying slightly different things, but as a group they feel intrusive and controlling and can set off our need for autonomy. This is also amplified by all the other messages we receive about how we 'should be' living our lives.

Here are some of the messages I currently feel bombarded with:

- Don't let you children have more than two hours of screen time a day.
- Don't have more than two hours of screen time yourself outside of work time.
- Wear sunscreen every day so you don't get skin cancer.
- Spend fifteen minutes a day in the sun without sunscreen so you get enough Vitamin D.
- Eat five serves of vegetables a day.
- Eat two serves of fruit a day.
- Drink alcohol in moderation (some health campaigns).
- Don't drink alcohol at all (other campaigns).
- Eat wholegrain cereals daily.
- Eat low GI foods.
- Eat breakfast.
- Eat regularly to keep your blood sugar levels even.

- Have a Pap smear.
- Check your breasts for lumps.
- Walk 10,000 steps a day.
- Get your heart rate up for at least an hour a week.
- Exercise for thirty minutes three times a week.
- Don't smack your children.
- Set boundaries with your children.
- Spend quality time with your children.
- Cook meals every day.
- Cook healthy snacks for the children's lunchbox.
- Buy local produce.
- Recycle, Reuse, Reduce.
- Ban plastic bags.
- Clean and floss your teeth daily.
- Go to the dentist.
- Have fish oil.
- Drive safely.
- Don't get road rage.
- Don't bully.

- Don't let others bully.
- Don't drink and drive.
- Meditate for an hour a day.
- Monitor yourself for depression.
- Monitor others for depression.
- Sleep at least seven hours a night.
- Resolve conflict through good communication.
- Monitor your children's internet usage.
- See all people as potential paedophiles.
- Keep your children safe.
- Let your children take risks.
- Stay positive, even when life is shit.
- Don't age.
- Get Botox.
- Hide grey hair.
- Wax everything off.
- Be sexy.
- Find some time for yourself.

And this list wasn't even hard to write! So, what happens as a result of the barrage of 'should'? Rebellion. I'll be damned,

Gen Y, if I am going to pour hot wax all over my body on a regular basis and rip all my body hair out! And two hours of screen time a day, does anyone actually *manage* that? And I'll eat five vegetables a day if you come over and cook them for me and make them interesting. As for alcohol, I'll listen to the advice I happen to prefer, thank you very much. And if you turn up on television with your bouncy ponytail and tell me your quick fitness tips, you will get a pillow thrown at your image. You just will. And I think I'm pretty normal in my reaction.

Let's just go through some of the implications of what I am saying when it comes to our weight:

- The more times we are told we must lose weight, the more likely we will decide we don't want to lose weight.

- The more messages we hear about healthy eating and exercising, the more likely we are to sit on the lounge and eat a bag of crisps.

- The more times we are shamed about our weight, the more likely we are to assert our autonomy by refusing to lose weight.

- The more times our partner rolls their eyes when we eat a bowl of ice-cream, the more likely we are to have seconds.

- The more times people try to 'help' or 'encourage' or 'inspire' us to lose weight, the more likely we are to become enraged, irrational people who throw cushions at well-intentioned bouncy girls on the television.

Am I making myself clear?

Now, of course, there is a problem here, because we don't want our autonomy reaction to make us put on more weight or sabotage our genuine efforts! We don't want to rebel so much that we do the opposite of what we genuinely desire and value. As I mentioned, every time that advertisement comes on asking me to think about my relationship with alcohol, I want to pour myself a glass of wine. But I *don't*. Because I know the only reason I want to do that is to rebel against the message. So, I will stop myself and ask, 'Do I genuinely want to have a glass of wine?' And often the answer is 'No'. I have learnt to firstly notice the reaction and then ignore it. This doesn't mean I am able to do this all the time. Our subconscious is very powerful and it will lead us astray at times, even against our better judgement. Don't let these messages get the better of you. If you are able to pushback without sabotaging yourself, do so. Say to yourself, 'I'll be damned if I am going to eat that pizza just because that doctor said I couldn't!' Rebel in a different way, and know that anything you are doing is just normal motivation at work.

CHAPTER 8

Personality

'A man should not strive to eliminate his complexes, but to get in accord with them; they are legitimately what directs his conduct in the world'

— Sigmund Freud

My desk at work is always messy. I have an administration officer, Carrie, whose desk at the end of the day is always spotless. It is so tidy, it actually looks like nobody works there. There have been many times in my life when I have tried to 'get organised' and have a tidier desk. This however has never, ever happened in more than twenty years of various jobs. I'm starting to think the problem is me!

I am not a lazy person. If I am passionate about something, I can work myself into the ground. In fact, I have done this several times in my life! When I am passionate about what I do I have a terrible habit of taking too much on, and this has never been good for my health! I am trying hard to reform myself out of this unfortunate habit though. It seems that I am not passionate about tidiness and have no trouble avoiding it. I now embrace this messy work environment as being 'my style'. I have a very creative mind and tend to get distracted from one project to the next. In my enthusiasm for my work projects, the task of keeping everything organised seems dull and unnecessary. I also like to have the key projects right at my fingertips—if I put them away, I literally struggle to find them.

Carrie, on the other hand, clearly functions better in an organised space. She has everything labelled and in a particular spot. To me, her work environment is sterile; to her it is calming. This is not something either of us chose, it sits deep within the core of who we are as people. No matter how often I have tried to use willpower to be neater, I have always failed. Luckily for me, I now have someone who completely compensates for my lack of motivation in this area!

Personality is something we recognise as being stable across our lifespan, and it consists of a set of characteristics or traits we have as individuals. Many of us know people who are 'stubborn' or 'excitable' or 'reserved' by nature. These things all fit into our personality. There are quite a number of different theories about personality, but the one I found most prominent in my reading was called the 'Big Five Personality Traits' (or the Five Factor Model) developed by researchers Robert McCrae and Oliver John. This model identified five key personality traits, and each individual sits on a scale for each of those traits. People can be on the 'high end' of the scale, meaning they have a lot of that trait. They can be on the 'low end' of the scale, meaning they have the opposite of that trait. Or they can be somewhere in the middle of the scale, expressing a more moderate version of the trait. The five personality traits identified in the model include the following:

1. *Conscientiousness*—people on the high end of conscientiousness are organised (like my administration officer), self-disciplined and tend to like things to be planned and goal focused. People on the low end of the conscientiousness scale might be messy (like me) and are more comfortable with change, spontaneity and flexibility.

2. *Agreeableness*—people high in agreeableness are compassionate and friendly, as well as trusting. They are generally well-tempered people. On the other end of the agreeableness scale are people who are argumentative, cynical and less trusting of others. They also have a tendency to get angry easily.

3. *Emotional Stability*—the high end of the scale refers to people who are calm and confident in nature and manage negative emotions with greater ease. At the low end of the scale are people who worry a lot and experience negative emotions more easily. They are more likely to experience anxiety and depression, and can be perceived as insecure.

4. *Openness to experience*—those on the high end of this scale enjoy creativity, emotion and new ideas. They enjoy adventure and different experiences. At the other end of the scale are people who are more likely to have pragmatic personalities, and like fulfilment to be gained through hard work and perseverance.

5. *Extroversion*—extroverts are those who are energetic and sociable. They tend to seek out stimulation and can be very talkative. At the other end of the scale is intro-

version. Introverts are more likely to be reserved and reflective by nature, and enjoy time to themselves.

Extroversion and introversion are the personality traits we hear the most about. An extrovert cannot 'will' themselves to be an introvert. It is embedded within their persona. I am an introvert by nature, although not at the extreme end. It is one of the reasons I am able to spend hours of my time writing. An extrovert would get bored and seek more social stimulation. And of course, I have always been an introvert. When my mother talks about me as a child, apparently I spent hours alone in my bedroom playing Lego or Barbies.

It has taken me years to realise that I am introvert, and that an essential aspect of this trait is the need to be alone on a regular basis. This allows me to recover and rejuvenate my energy supplies. Motherhood and introversion are therefore not a great match, because for at least a decade you are NEVER ALONE—not even in the bathroom. Add fulltime work into this scenario and you have a real problem. Again, this is a life lesson I have had to learn the hard way by reaching the exhaustion point a number of times in my life. I need time and space to regain energy. And I'm pretty sure no one considered the needs of introverts when they designed open plan office spaces! Even small amounts of time alone can be health enhancing for an introvert.

Now, of course, introversion doesn't mean that I don't enjoy socialising. In fact, I love people! But time with people has to be balanced out with time alone. And if I am feeling run down, the need to be alone becomes the higher priority. After a particularly bad bout of exhaustion, I actually had to cut back my work hours in order to get the space and time that I needed for my health. As a mother who is also a carer and worker, the exhaustion was completely and utterly debilitating. I just had to accept the fact that I needed to build in time for myself if I was going to be healthy. Thankfully an understanding manager also recognised reducing my hours was in my best interests. As an introvert, I am seem also attracted to fitness activities that I do alone. I like walking the dog, yoga and swimming—all solitary and peaceful forms of activity. I enjoy exercise far more when it also gives me some time to myself.

Personality traits and their connection to weight management have been an interesting area to explore further. While I'm sure my introverted personality has a lot to do with the exercise choices I make, I didn't find any research specifically related to the topic. However, I did find some studies that looked at personality traits and weight. While they were sparse in nature, they were compelling to read. The most robust study was conducted by Angelina Sutin and her colleagues. They examined data from a fifty-year aging study and looked at personality traits in relationship to weight, and weight fluctuations over the lifespan.

They found that people high in the personality trait of conscientiousness were more likely to be thin across their lifespan. People high in this trait are organised and enjoy rigid routines and rituals. My ultimate test on extreme conscientiousness is the clothes peg test. You'll be amazed by how many people need to use matching clothes pegs when hanging out their washing. By this I mean, each item of clothing needs to have clothes pegs that are matching in design and colour. I find this completely bizarre! As long as the pegs keep the clothes attached to the line, I really don't see a problem. But I know people who will go outside and change the pegs if someone else has hung out the washing and the pegs do not match. I also know of people who have to match the colour of the pegs to the colour of the item of clothing they are hanging out. Now of course, we can all see that it makes no real difference what pegs people use when they hang out their washing, but you'd be amazed by how many people need to match the pegs. Extremely conscientious people just feel better when the pegs match. Maybe they are thinner because of all that walking outside to ensure the pegs match!

My husband has a conscientious personality, although not of the clothes peg matching variety. He does, however, tend to do the exact same thing at the exact same time each week. Every Sunday evening, he cuts up a large container of raw vegetables to take to work for snacks throughout the week. He does this without fail. He also has a very specific exercise regime, with certain activities on certain days of the week. If he misses a session, he makes up for it at another time. Not surprisingly, the study found that people with a conscientious personality were the ones with the most stable weight pattern over their lifespan. They didn't have weight fluctuations in which they gained or lost large amounts of weight. We all know people with a conscientious personality type, and you can see how this trait helps them with their weight.

A rigid exercise regime would never work for me. As a less conscientious person, I am far more distracted by my mood and feelings on the day. I like exercise, but the type of exercise I do will often be determined by the weather or my mood. On a hot day, I like to jump in the pool and have a swim. If the weather is balmy, I am down by the ocean with the dog going for a walk. If the music is on at home, I find myself dancing around the kitchen and having fun with my daughter. A beautiful sunrise inspires me to do yoga. I don't have 'exercise days' or specific 'exercise times'. I enjoy a more flexible routine. As a result though, I am far less reliable when it comes to exercising. The study demonstrated that people like me, with a more flexible approach to routine, gain more weight over their life. Good news!

I seem to have passed on my lack of conscientiousness to my daughter, Maya. Her bedroom has always been extremely messy. Peter and I have done all the regular things to try and get her to be tidier. We've nagged, we've begged, we've used incentives and we've set punishments. In one particularly determined period, Peter would take her into her room and together they would tidy for ten minutes each evening. After a week, the room was looking quite neat and Peter said to her, 'Is it nice having a tidy room?' She replied, 'Not really. It's just not a current priority for me.' She was nine years old! Sometimes kids know themselves better than adults. And, of course, she was spot-on. It's not in her nature to want to have a tidy room. Her lack of conscientiousness meant she had a relaxed attitude when it came to tidiness. Peter and I had that moment where we had to consider: 'How much do we battle this?' The constant focus on her messy room was not making the household happy. It felt like most of our conversations with her were focused on this one negative topic. So, we decided to let it go for a while and just shut the door when it bothered us. Our one rule was there was to be no food in her room. And yes, it got worse before it got better. Slowly though, she started to do small things to keep her room in a better condition. This seemed to occur as a result of growing up rather than any tough parenting strategy we used. At the end of the day, we decided not to argue over something that clearly wasn't in her nature. It seemed she couldn't help it any more than I could help my messy desk! I hate it when your children turn out just like you!

So as a person low on conscientiousness, I am more likely to gain weight, but as an introvert there is a little bit of hope for me because the study found that people high in extroversion were the ones more likely to gain weight. Extroverts need stimulation on a regular basis, and it is theorised that they may do this by seeking out food. Extroverts therefore could be the people we call 'boredom eaters'. As sociable types, I would also suggest they are more likely to spend time in environments that serve food and alcohol. Extroverts can't bear to be alone for any length of time. My friend Kym, the foodie, is an extrovert. She eats hard and she exercises hard—but always with a group of people around her. Because she lived alone she would go out four or five times a week to eat. But she'd also exercise at least that many times too. And some of her exercise rituals were quite bizarre. She once pushed a car up a hill with a group of friends as an exercise challenge! She's also one of those people who will do exercise events all night, and she's been known to climb a major mountain or two. You may have guessed that, along with extroversion, she has a large dose of conscientiousness. Sometimes I felt exhausted just listening to how much Kym could fit into one day! 'When are you ever still?' I'd ask her. That's an extrovert for you though. Apparently, their big personalities also come with a big appetite. Extroverts were found to binge drink and overeat more often too. Don't feel bad for the extroverts though, because other studies also show they are happier. These really are the fat and happy people of the world!

Let's move onto the trait of disagreeableness. I'm not sure anyone in my life would like to be identified as being disagreeable in nature, but I certainly know a few! Just the other day I heard two grown women have an argument about eating in the office. One complained about the smelly food her colleague was eating. The colleague eating the smelly food then complained about the sound of the crunchy carrots the other often ate. The complaining deteriorated into a verbal showdown from there. I was sitting at my desk thinking, 'Really'? Not only did they raise their own stress, they raised the stress of the entire office as we all ducked for cover to ensure we didn't inadvertently get involved. So I'm just saying that some people have a pretty low tolerance for anything they find irritating!

The office is always an interesting place to observe different personality types. People being in close proximity for hours each day can be volatile. Here are some things I have found bizarre about office behaviour. I once heard a woman come out of the bathroom completely outraged that someone had not changed the toilet paper roll. She was determined to discover who the 'culprit' was and to shame them for their behaviour. I have heard adults argue over who owns a desk chair and who moved it. I have seen people berate others because their voices were too loud on the phone. I have heard adults tell other adults they are laughing too much and need to be quiet. And I once received an email from a colleague because I apparently closed a door too loudly. So yes, disagreeableness is definitely a thing.

Apart from the fact that disagreeableness makes workplaces tense and frustrating at times, the study found that people who were low on the agreeableness trait gained more weight. The theory was that people who get angry and frustrated easily also have more frequent spikes in their cortisol levels. This spike in cortisol levels also lasts longer. Cortisol is a hormone connected to stress. It is part of a response called 'fight or flight' which has an important purpose for survival. Unfortunately people with a disagreeable nature are triggering this response when the toilet roll has not been replaced as opposed to when they are in real danger! And the response is more significant and longer lasting than for those people who have a more agreeable personality. Cortisol is well known for being connected to weight gain, and in particular weight gain around our internal organs (that is, on our stomachs). I explain the fight or flight response in a little more detail in the chapter on instinct, but for now it is enough to know that this response makes us eat and makes us gain weight. That is why I am always supportive of a person under high stress saying they want to eat cake. They are literally craving something from an instinctual level. This is not something that is easily battled through willpower! Unfortunately for people with a disagreeable personality trait this happens more often and with greater severity. I wonder what would happen if we told them, 'Calm down. You're making yourself fat!' I'm not sure it would go down well. So perhaps there are fat and cranky people, as well as fat and happy people in the world!

The personality trait of emotional stability can also have a big impact on workplace dynamics. I once worked with a woman we described as 'the tornado'. When she entered a room, her energy seemed to take over. She talked fast and loud, and there was always a dramatic story that seemed to be of life or death importance to tell. She would then swoop out of the room as fast as she came in. Everyone would take a deep breath and try to regain the peaceful environment that had existed before she arrived. Her energy literally felt like a tornado that came, caused chaos, and left again. People low in emotional stability struggle to regulate their emotions. They can have amazing highs and dramatic lows. The unfortunate thing is that they often pull the people working with them up or down with the drama as well. We all know people that are offended by the smallest comment, who hold a grudge that can go on for years, who need an hour to debrief after one poorly worded email. Being unstable emotionally can also lead to extreme patterns of weight-related behaviour. In the study, they were more likely to weight cycle or have significant weight fluctuations over their lifespan. And they also tended to experience more extreme weight patterns at both the low end (under-eating) and the high end (over-eating).

When people are emotionally unstable, they may use food (or the control of food) as a way to help them regulate how they feel. After all, food can give us a sense of comfort and safety. Those who experience more extreme emotions may seek out this sense of regulation through food. Emotional instability may also be related to other impulsive behaviours such as shopping, drinking or even violence. Impulsivity was the component of emotional stability most linked to weight gain, with those high in impulsivity showing a weight of about eleven kilograms higher than those low on impulsivity. People who are emotionally unstable could also have more issues related to self-esteem. As a result, negative comments and messages from the world around them may have a greater impact, and in fact add to their weight problem. Another study examined body image and weight over a ten-year period in adolescents. Those who had poor body image gained more weight over the ten years than those who felt good about their bodies. This happened despite what they weighed at the beginning of the study. Weight gain was also linked to how much the parents worried about the child's weight and focused on it as an issue.

I find it interesting when I see people write or comment on people who are overweight in the media or in fashion. Recently, a *Sports Illustrated* fashion show included women who were not the average stick-thin models. I noted that quite a few media people questioned the wisdom of this, suggesting that it would normalise obesity and increase the problem. But I believe that the complete opposite is true, and the study mentioned above supports my theory. When people who are different in shapes and sizes are visible to the community, and even linked to beauty and desirability, people feel better about themselves. Feeling good about ourselves puts us in a more stable position motivationally and encourages or inspires us to take care of ourselves rather than punish ourselves. And surely a fashion show is there to sell clothes. Clothes need to be suitable for all kinds of bodies, not just thin bodies. I saw the same debate occur recently when a store dared to have mannequins for their lingerie that were a size sixteen. Given a size sixteen is an average woman's body size, I think it is reasonable to demonstrate to these perfectly normal women that there is lingerie that fits them! The average person is likely to be positively motivated by these images. And for someone who is more emotionally unstable, it may be even more important. What seems logical is in fact completely wrong—people who feel good about themselves are more motivated to be healthy, not the other way around!

Personality definitely has an impact on motivation and behaviours related to weight management. Now, of course, our personality is actually a combination of all of these traits mixed together to varying degrees. Most people are not at the extreme ends of any of these traits. Peter is conscientious, but he doesn't need to match his pegs. I am introverted, but I love spending time with people. Personality doesn't change much over a person's lifetime, so again, we need to accept what we have when it comes to the influence of our personality on our motivation for weight management. Knowing our traits might help us to manage them more effectively, or perhaps reduce some of the negative consequences. At the end of the day though, I'm still going to have a messy desk at work, and I'm never going to stick to a rigid exercise regime. It seems that my administration officer is just going to have to take a deep breath to manage her stress levels when it comes to my chaos. Sorry Carrie!

CHAPTER 9

Instinct

'In art, as in love, instinct is enough'

— Anatole France

My dog Coco is like a child to me. Part of me wanted to have another baby—I got a dog instead. Despite having watched the *Dog Whisperer with Cesar Millan* for years, I did everything wrong when it came to my dog. I allowed her to jump on the sofa, I gave her food from the table, she slept on my children's beds, she barked at the neighbours and she walked ahead of me on the lead. So, I'm really sorry, Cesar, I failed doggy 101. But in all honesty, I didn't really care. I treated her like a baby and it made me happy. Because she was so cute and so embedded within our human lives, it was easy at times to forget that she was in fact a dog. One day she brought this home to us in a moment of startling reality.

Maya and I were walking her at the local park, a lush green space with plenty of shade and tropical plants. Coco was (as usual) leading the way and letting us know where she wanted to go for a sniff. At one point she took us to a group of low-lying shrubs and went in deep to explore further. She was quite adamant about this particular location and in fact refused to move on after a number of minutes. Getting bored, I pulled her lead quite hard to force her out of the bushes. She emerged with something in her mouth that I couldn't quite make out. I then heard my daughter gasp and watched as she stepped back in complete horror, hand over her mouth. It was at this point I realised what was wedged between the jaws of my beloved, cute, human-like hound: a bird. And not just any bird, but a rainbow lorikeet, one of the most beautiful-looking birds you can imagine. The blood drained from my face as I realised my gorgeous dog was in fact a cold-hearted bird-killing beast! I managed to tug her hard enough that she lost grip and, despite her protestations, we dragged Coco away from her treasure. We now refer to this as 'The Incident of 2016'. Maya couldn't talk to the dog for a week. I also felt a little distant and confused. How could this pretty little dog who loved smoked salmon, belly rubs and lazing on the sofa be the same animal that killed a defenceless and beautiful bird? We felt traumatised. But of course, we were the ones being ridiculous. Coco was full of instincts that didn't disappear simply because I treated her like a human and fed her triple cream brie. She was bred to hunt. And she hunted.

Human beings assume they have outgrown instinct as a motivating force in their behaviours. As I was writing this book, my administration officer, Carrie, decided to go on a diet. In her drawer, she had sachets of soup mix, which she was 'allowed' to have as snacks. She was also weighing everything she ate so she could put her body into a state of 'ketosis' as per the diet guidelines. I tried to be neutral, neither encouraging the diet nor criticising it, but, as I watched her, my little heart was breaking. One morning she was ravenous. She had already had the special little soup snack and was still hungry, so she decided to eat her lunch early—it was a sparse-looking salad with a small portion of low-fat meat. After eating this as well, she declared, 'I'm still hungry'. Trying yet again to be neutral, I said nothing. It was only 11.30 am and she wouldn't be 'allowed' to have another delightful-looking soup sachet for a number of hours. She tried to distract herself with tasks, but within half an hour she went and bought a hot chocolate and a chocolate muffin. I wanted to wrap her in my arms and say, 'It's not your fault!' I'm sure she had an internal dialogue through the afternoon in which she chastised herself for her 'lack of willpower'. Meanwhile, my internal dialogue was harping, 'I have to get this book written so people stop torturing themselves!'

Here was an incredibly self-disciplined woman. Super-organised and diligent, she was a master of administration. But she couldn't fight intense hunger with willpower! And neither can you. Eating is an instinct. We are meant to eat. Our entire genetic make-up is designed to help us survive, and that means eating. Instincts are described as behaviours humans have that are not taught, but are somehow 'known' through our genes. Instincts are present in all humans and across all races. We all laugh, we all smile, we all cry, we all sleep and we all eat. These are all instinctual behaviours. While we like to think we have learnt to control our instincts, watching Carrie eat her chocolate muffin, I'm thinking we still have a way to go with this as a species! We didn't evolve from a group of people who had supermarkets and a plentiful supply of food. We evolved from hunter-gatherers who sought specific nutritional items for survival. Despite the fact we now shop in sterile environments with shopping trolleys, we still have the same instincts.

We now know scientifically that different foods contain different nutrients, and that these different nutrients sustain us and support our health. Our hunter-gatherer ancestors did not have textbooks to inform them of this fact. Instead, they had tastebuds. The original purpose of tastebuds was to ensure that humans ate the things they needed to in order to get variety in their diet. It also stopped them from eating things that were potentially poisonous. Therefore, human beings were driven through instinct to eat salty, sweet and fatty foods, and we still are. These flavours taste good to us and we are drawn to eating them.

And let's face it, eating is *fun*! When we eat things that taste good, we generate a dopamine reaction. Dopamine is a neurotransmitter (or a chemical in the brain) that moves between brain cells and transmits information. A release of dopamine provides a sense of pleasure and therefore motivationally encourages us to do more of that behaviour. Researchers have studied the effectiveness of dopamine receptors in mice. (In brain cells, dopamine receptors absorb the dopamine.) The researchers found that when the receptors are reduced, the mice stop eating and starve themselves to death. Therefore, food is meant to give us a sense of pleasure (via dopamine) so that we keep eating and keep ourselves alive! While I was researching for this book, I also came across information that indicated that some people who overeat may have problems with their dopamine receptors, causing them to keep seeking dopamine by eating more food. The biological basis for eating is not equal across the human population!

The plentiful supply of inexpensive food has also helped create a culture of over-eaters. Instinctually, we are driven to prepare for times of famine. This of course was inevitable when we lived in nomadic tribes. And yet, the instinct to eat more calories than are required for daily energy requirements still appears to be present. Studies have shown that we tend to eat whatever food is in front of us. So, large serving sizes lead to large consumption. However, rather than resulting from a 'lack of willpower', much of this over-eating pattern is likely to come from this instinct. Nature developed a very effective system called adipose tissue (or fat deposits) to ensure we had a plentiful supply of energy in case famine hit. In fact, people who gain weight easily are considered to be advanced, from an evolutionary perspective! Small comfort for those who gain weight just at the smell of food!

Serving sizes are completely out of control. And who is to blame? Was it the generation of 'all you can eat' buffet restaurants that exploded during the eighties and nineties? Was it the soft drink companies that competed to have the biggest bottle? Was it the nannas of the world that forced us to eat everything on our plates? Was it the platter-sized dinner plates that started showing up in restaurants and then eventually our homes? Was it the super-sizing culture in fast food restaurants, chocolate manufacture and muffin baking? Or was it our own need to feel like we were getting a bargain? And the truth is we are all to blame for this ridiculous over-consuming culture on some level. But our human instinct to consume and create energy stores is also to blame. The community created the over-eating culture and the community will need to work towards unravelling it, because we cannot expect the motivational drive from instinct to suddenly disappear.

I remember a time when our family of five would share one large serve of fries when we ate takeaway. I remember the children being forced to share a soft drink with each other. I remember Nana baking cakes that were the size of a plum, not an orange. Is the 'value meal' killing is? Value for money but not for health? These are the hard questions we have to ask as a community, but they are necessary reflections.

When Carrie said she was on a diet to put her body into ketosis, what that meant was that she was putting her body into a position where it would have to use her fat supplies for energy. That all sounds very easy, but the body was not designed to give up these fat supplies easily. Biologically, we are driven to function from carbohydrate sources. That is what our muscles and brain prefer. Our fat stores can be converted, but this takes additional energy. As a result, our body urges us to eat more carbohydrates, because it is trying to keep our fat stores intact. That is the moment we go and buy a chocolate muffin. Our body is literally yearning for a hit of carbs! Instinct takes over our behaviour, and it says, 'eat carbs you damn fool!'

I have tried to eat salad and a low-fat protein for lunch, which seems to be the current trend. I have now done it often enough that I know the outcome. If I eat my lunch at midday, I feel reasonably satisfied for a short period of time. However, by two pm I am starving. Subway cookies, not to mention cronuts, are within metres of my office door. If I eat salad for lunch, I feast on all sorts of delightful sweet things to get through the afternoon. What happens if I eat a lunch that includes some carbohydrates? I get through the afternoon on a cup of tea. This pattern has been so consistent, I don't even bother with the salad for lunch anymore. It actually makes my eating worse, not better. That is the thing about instinct, good intentions go out the window. And so, motivationally, I know I am actually better eating carbohydrates and maintaining better control over my eating.

Many of my colleagues have also discovered I am the go-to person if they want to justify their stress eating. A bad email, a tough meeting or an inconsiderate phone call and they come flocking to my desk saying, 'I need chocolate'. I will always be supportive of this 'need'. Most of us know that stress makes us want to eat and there is an instinctual basis to this desire.

Stress, as mentioned earlier, is really a physiological response called 'fight or flight'. It is a survival mechanism in which blood rushes to our major muscle groups and away from 'unnecessary' functions (at least temporarily unnecessary) such as our digestive system. We start sweating, our heart rate and breathing increase, our vision narrows and we become deeply alert. It is a very quick and effective system if we come across a snake, are attacked unexpectedly or a car is about to run us over. It is a poor mechanism if we are reading an upsetting email. The whole purpose of the system is to ensure we can quickly react to danger and MOVE. This requires us to use up our resources and energy supplies. Our body assumes that, because we have had the stress reaction, we have used up valuable energy. Once the reaction settles, it drives an instinct in us to resupply the energy supplies. And the preference to recoup those supplies comes through calorie-dense foods with plenty of rich fats and easy-to-use carbohydrates. That sounds a lot like chocolate doesn't it? Or cheesecake perhaps?

In fact, it seems that, when we are stressed, the food we eat is more likely to be converted to fat supplies because of a release of the hormone cortisol which we discussed earlier. The more stressed we are, the more we eat, and the main weight we gain is from that food we consume in that moment. How many people do you know who live in a state of chronic stress? I look around and all I see are people rushing, fretting and feeling like they are failing. They are working and studying and caring for children. They are exercising and shopping and mowing lawns. All while being under a huge amount of stress.

So I think we need to ask ourselves an important question: how much is stress contributing to the obesity epidemic? What percentage could be reduced or managed just from a change in our stress levels? And if it's significant, what we would need to change to ensure our lives were less stressful? Would it require shorter working weeks? Better child care systems? Cheaper housing? Reduced out-of-school activities? Effective aged care services? Free yoga and meditation classes? What would it require to take the pressure down a few notches to allow people a moment to breathe? While complex, I do not think these are unsolvable issues. There is no switch to turn off the instinctual fight-and-flight response. We must acknowledge its benefits and work more effectively with the challenges it creates in current environments. If we are stressed, we will not only eat more but gain more weight as a result.

There may be some good news when it comes to the motivational forces of instinct though. We also have an instinct to *move*. Anyone who has raised a child will know how pointless it is trying to get a toddler to stay still. Once they learn to move, they don't want to stop. They are too damn excited about their new skills and too curious about their worlds to sit still for any length of time. But then, what do we tend to do with this innate need to move? We spend the next few years trying to get rid of it! 'Sit still'. 'Stay still'. 'Stop moving'. These are all statements a child hears thousands of times in their first few years. In fact, the children who struggle to stay still are labelled as 'naughty'. We do it in schools, in church, in restaurants, at the movies, at the dinner table, in front of visitors and anywhere else. And after years and years of this what happens? Children end up sitting still—for hours and hours on end. We have literally socialised the movement out of them. Because kids who move are kids who get in trouble.

Movement is natural and very important. Occupational therapists who work with children know that movement is a form of arousal. It stimulates the nervous system and enables it to stay 'awake' and 'alert'. This level of alertness in our nervous system supports our ability to concentrate, to solve problems and to learn. Have you ever spent an entire day in a workshop or lecture? Have you looked around the room and noticed what is actually happening? People will be doodling, rocking, fidgeting, tapping their feet, chewing their pens and a range of other small movements. When we are forced to sit still for long periods of time, we struggle to stay alert. To keep our nervous system 'awake', we have to do small things to try and increase our arousal levels. It actually helps us to focus on the content of the workshop. Without this movement, we would all start to become drowsy. However, in these situations we have been trained that only small, discrete movements are acceptable. Movement is an instinctive sensory need that helps us to function.

When we spend time moving, we are able to spend time in focused attention. This need seems to be more extreme in people with autism or other disabilities, and that is why the focus has generally been on this part of the population. You can now buy chairs that have movement built into them so children with autism can move their legs, rock back and forth or swing for periods of time when sitting at their desks at school. Their natural need to move is starting to be accommodated. But the reality is we all have an instinctive need for movement. This need has been made socially unacceptable. Given the current obesity epidemic, the notion of movement as being rude or impolite needs to be reversed. Even small movements accommodated across the day can help with our health and wellbeing. I'm sure we have amazing designers who can create new environments in schools and workplaces that create and inspire movement, rather than hinder it.

I'd also like to see our communities really re-embrace the idea of dance. In times gone by, dancing was a common social event and form of celebration. Most cultures around the world have used music and dance. To me, this indicates there is something deeply instinctive about it. Dance seems to have a meaning that resonates within our souls. It energises people and brings them joy. It also connects us with other human beings, which is another instinctual need. As I've been bringing myself out of this period of hopelessness and towards better health, I have started bringing more music back into my life. The music inherently brings me joy, but it also brings movement. Whether I am ironing or cooking or just hanging out, with music on I tend to be moving. It can be anything from tapping my foot, clapping my hands, to outright dancing. It is an effortless form of movement. I am not thinking about it and I don't have to use any willpower. Maybe instead of telling people they need to exercise more, we just need to tell them to put music on more often!

When it comes to motivation and instinct, there are elements that can help us and elements that can hinder us when it comes to weight management. Eating so little that you become ravenously hungry is not likely to help you. Dancing and laughing with your children though is something that could. If we carefully redesigned our communities to embrace movement and decrease stress, we could significantly affect the obesity issues we face. A small decrease in some of our serving sizes also wouldn't hurt!

CHAPTER 10

Intuition

'Intuition is a spiritual faculty and does not explain, but simply points the way'

— Florence Scovel Shinn

Some theorists put instinct and intuition into the same category, but for me they are quite different. Instinct to me is more about behaviour whereas intuition is a level of consciousness or a sense of 'knowing'. Some say that intuition derives from previous experience, but that seems like a shallow explanation from my perspective. The research on intuition and its impact on motivation is essentially non-existent, but in my experience it is a deeply embedded component of our motivational drive. I could go on to theorise about where intuition comes from and why it exists, but, at best, it would be an academic discussion. It doesn't matter why or how it exists, just that it does. I'm sure a room full of people would all have differing opinions anyway, so you can use any framework that feels comfortable and familiar to you.

When I was feeling depressed and hopeless, I was gaining weight and I knew it. But I also knew it wasn't the time to worry about my weight. That feeling came from my intuition. There was a sense I needed to be kind to myself and to ride out the feelings. It was like my intuition was telling me, 'You're doing a good job. Don't add any extra pressure right now'. It would have been easy to ignore this intuition and add another psychological burden onto myself—the burden of self-criticism and guilt about my weight. But intuition protected me from going down that path.

My life is the equivalent of universal boot camp. I feel like I am in the fast class for spiritual growth and development, and my son is the head teacher. I don't say this lightly. I truly believe his purpose in the world is to teach. And the first thing he taught me was to pay attention to my intuition. Having a child that doesn't do things like other children means that you quickly learn the normal rules and information on parenting don't apply. That leaves you with only one source of good information—your gut feeling. The first few years of listening to intuition took some practice. This was a period where I frequently experienced doubt about my intuition. As a result, I would look for reassurance from it over and over again. One of the amazing things about intuition I discovered through this process was that it was deeply consistent. Strategies such as problem-solving often led to different answers at different times, but intuition always said the same thing. Eventually it won me over so much I now won't make any decision unless my intuition confirms it.

When I say 'listen' to my intuition, what I really mean is to 'feel' it. Intuition for me is often a body-based sensation. If I get myself into a calm and relaxed state, my body literally 'talks' to me through the sensations I experience. A very calm and confident feeling in my stomach indicates that my thought is on the right track. A tumultuous feeling means absolutely not. A 'non-feeling' (that is, neither a strong positive nor a strong negative feeling) is also a no or 'it isn't important'. Once you have learnt to listen and use intuition as your decision-maker, you will never go back. It is far too reliable! I find other people to-and-fro when it comes to making major life decisions. They feel anxious, overwhelmed or torn by the options. I just find my calmness and listen closely. It takes a lot of stress out of life!

There are many people in the world who have a finely honed sense of intuition. They may have grown up in a culture that teaches children from a young age to focus on intuition, they may have come to it through life experiences like I have, or perhaps they have read books or taken classes to try and learn more about it. How does intuition relate to motivation though?

I sometimes reflect on the story of one of my best friends, Emma, and her husband, Tim. He felt really 'unfit' and went to many doctors complaining of breathlessness and exhaustion. Medical opinion suggested he was just unfit and kept encouraging him to exercise and improve his fitness. He followed their suggestions but nothing improved. Tim kept going back to doctors and they kept giving him the same suggestions. This went on for four years. No matter how much he tried to exercise, the breathlessness and fatigue remained.

Now you can imagine how motivated he felt to exercise during this period! He was experiencing *extreme* fatigue and breathlessness. Exhausted and disillusioned with the medical practitioners he had been seeing, Tim eventually found a GP who told him they would keep searching until they found the answer to his health problems. Eventually they discovered he had something called 'pulmonary hypertension'. Far from being a relief though, this diagnosis came with a terminal prognosis. Tim was dying and there was nothing anyone could do to stop it. He passed away at the age of twenty-six. Tim and Emma had hoped that a heart-lung transplant might extend his life for a period, but Tim never made it to the transplant stage. Tim and Emma's intuition told them something was seriously wrong with Tim. No amount of exercise was ever going to help, and yet it would have been easy to label Tim as 'unmotivated'.

Tim was a thin man, but I once saw a television story of a young woman who was overweight and was eventually diagnosed with the same condition. Because of her weight, everyone from doctors to teachers drove her to exercise and told her she was breathless because of her weight issues. At one point, she struggled to walk up a set of stairs and was berated by a teacher for being lazy in front of her class. But she wasn't lazy, she was dying. Both her and her mother felt there was something wrong, but yet again their intuition was ignored for many years. I don't know what happened to this young lady, but I hope she was able to beat the odds and live for a long time.

As a therapist, I have learnt to deeply respect people's intuition. It is a form of knowledge I have no access to. And so, if people tell me 'something doesn't feel right' or they 'don't think this is helping' or 'it's not the right time at the moment', I pay careful attention. Any expertise I carry must work with what the person's intuition is telling them. Again, people whose motivation says 'stop' or 'not now' can look like people who have poor motivation. From the outside, it can look like a series of excuses stopping them from making progress. And often, even the person themself does not understand why they feel 'stuck'. But once you start exploring what people's 'gut feeling' is saying, there is often a sense of something not being quite right.

We went through this ourselves when Evan was young and we were trying to toilet-train him. It was the year before he went to school and there was incredible pressure to try and get him toilet-trained before he started. We tolerated an entire year without pull-ups to try and 'get him toilet-trained'. After a year, we felt completely and utterly exhausted. We had dealt with endless toileting 'accidents' and all the washing and cleaning that came with it. After a year, our intuition told us that he couldn't feel when he needed to go. And just to prove my point, he is still not completely toilet-trained at fifteen. How much effort do you put into something when your gut is telling you it is not the right time? That is a journey that continues for us and we are now far more inclined to listen to our intuition.

When I was feeling depressed and hopeless, the time was not right to focus on my weight. And looking back, I now believe that time was something I needed. Sometimes I think we are in too much of a hurry to eliminate negative feelings. In fact, during that time, people suggested perhaps I should go and see a therapist. But I felt (intuitively) that a therapist wasn't going to be able to help me. And now, looking back, I can see that the time I took facilitated in me a very important process of deep acceptance. In mental health language, we might refer to this point as 'radical acceptance'. It was a place in which I stopped trying to solve the problem and just accepted the problem's existence. Radical acceptance is about accepting those things that seem completely unacceptable. For me, that was my son's violence. For others, it could be the murder of a family member, the abuse or neglect by a parent during childhood, or the persistence and pervasion of daily anxiety. There are many things we don't want to accept, but they still exist. And sometimes the effort of trying to make them go away is what actually causes the most pain.

Ironically, or perhaps profoundly, once I found a place of radical acceptance, my son's challenging behaviours significantly reduced. I now wonder if he sensed my energy or need to change him. Once I stopped doing that, and accepted the violence as part of him, the energy shifted. Autism is like an overly sensitive radio channel that reacts to all types of energy fields. So perhaps it was me making the problem worse all along.

In my own personal belief system, my intuition, often through my motivation, acts like a spiritual guide. If I am not motivated about something, I start asking the question, 'What is my gut telling me?' Earlier in the book, I discussed trying to write academic articles and feeling unmotivated. I now believe that my intuition was telling me that it wasn't the right pathway for me to take. My lack of motivation for the activity helped me to identify that this was the case. Logic told me, 'It's a good thing to do. It will give you credibility. It will look good on your CV'. And the people around me were telling me similar things. But my gut was telling me through my lack of motivation, 'Wrong way! Go back!' I am naturally inclined to be a storyteller, reflector and philosopher, not an academic. I now believe I am supposed to write books like this, not academic articles or texts. Perhaps the last thing the world needs is another academic. Maybe my purpose is to be more of a 'translator', someone who can take concepts from research and weave them into story. This book has been highly motivating to write, so that tells me I am doing what I should be doing.

I have just talked about my intuition and how helpful it is in my life. But remember, this was a skill I learnt. You can also start to connect more with your intuition—it just takes practice. This eventually leads to greater confidence in the intuitive process. I am not a great meditator, but when I am struggling to hear my intuition, I do go into a meditative state. This only takes a few minutes though, so don't think you need to spend hours meditating to listen to your gut. Sometimes I even do it while I am in the shower. All I do is take a couple if deep breaths, spend a moment feeling the water hit my body to bring me into mindfulness, and then just pay attention to my intuition. As I've said, I experience sensations in my gut, but I have also had random thoughts pop into my head at times. I take this all in as part of the intuitive process.

If you are struggling with your weight and you want to have a sense of where to go from here, start practising intuition and see what happens. Worst case scenario is that you will experience the benefits of deep breathing and a moment of mindfulness. Firstly, I would encourage you to listen to your intuition about strategies that will or won't work for you when it comes to weight management. What feels genuine and what feels like a sales pitch? Should you really consider medication or another program? In particular, pay attention if you are considering options like surgery. Is this something your intuition is telling you to do?

The timing of change may be important too. Intuition could be telling you the best place to start is with self-acceptance. Shame and self-loathing are never a good place from which to begin positive changes. I know this sounds airy-fairy, but honestly, seeing yourself as a valid and worthwhile person who deserves a good life, and deserves good health, is a much better place to begin a journey of change. Perhaps that needs to be the initial focus.

Your intuition could also give you answers to other questions. Is the problem bigger than weight? Do you need to focus on stress first? Are you grieving or going through a lot of change? Are you in a toxic relationship? Are you just trying to survive the day? Is there something underlying that's happening with your health? Are you living the life you are meant to be living? All these things may come through your intuition. If you have a strong gut feeling about something, stop and reflect.

It took me a decade of 'practising intuition' to become really confident and skilled in it. It is not a process that ends though. I am still building skills in this area and see it as a lifelong journey. One thing I know for sure though is that if my intuition says 'no', even if it seems illogical, I will not be motivated to progress. Anyone who tries to argue a point with my intuitive process is in for a battle they can't win, I'm afraid—even when that person is me!

SECTION 3

Shallow motivational drivers

CHAPTER 11

Attitudes and beliefs

*'People almost invariably arrive at their
beliefs not on the basis of proof,
but on the basis of what they find attractive'*

— Blaise Pascal

I used to believe that people who talked about intuition like I do now were bizarre. And then I experienced intuition myself and changed my mind. I used to believe I was doing a fantastic job as an occupational therapist. And then I learnt more about motivation and changed my mind. I used to believe that you could make children eat healthy food. And then I had children who refused to eat and changed my mind. Life has an interesting way of convincing us that things may not be what we thought or anticipated. I've had a range of beliefs over the years that I now think were completely and utterly wrong. I probably have beliefs right now that, in another decade, I will also think are wrong.

A belief is a principle or idea that is considered to be true or correct. An attitude is how we feel, think or react to a belief. I believe that it is wrong to smack children. Therefore, my attitude is one of distress when I hear of someone smacking a child. I believe that being gay is a normal human state. And therefore, my attitude is that gay people should have the same rights as heterosexual people. I believe that diets do not work. And my attitude is to feel sad and frustrated when people use them. The belief is a thought. The attitude includes the feeling related to the thought. It is absolutely true that beliefs and attitudes affect our motivation. But it is also true that they sit in a shallower space in our psychological onion. This is because they tend to change quite a bit over our lifetime.

We are all convinced that our beliefs are correct, until we start believing something else. There was a time in the world when slavery was thought to be reasonable, because it was written about in the Bible. That belief now seems absurd. There was a time when lobotomies were given as a legitimate medical treatment. Now this is seen as unethical and inhumane. There was a time when breastfeeding was considered inconvenient or even disgusting. Now it is seen as beautiful and a desirable option for the baby. It is hard to imagine there are beliefs we hold right now that we will look back on with dismay. But that is one of the few certainties in the world. Times change, and so do beliefs and attitudes.

Think about the community's beliefs and attitudes to weight over the years. Chubby women were once esteemed for their beauty. They were envied for their curves, and it was a sign of their wealth and their social class. I long for those days when paintings of women with large breasts, full arms, and rolls of stomach were held up as the ultimate beauty. I might have been an artist's model in those days! In medieval times, vegetables were considered food only suitable for animal consumption!

People lived on bread and meat broth, thrown down by a few glasses of beer or wine. Now we have guidelines about how many vegetables we should eat that even vegetarians struggle to consume. Baby boomers and generation X lived through the 'fat is bad' era and we all avoided eggs and avocados. Now we are eating avocados and eggs every day.

If we believed what we heard about weight management, we'd think all we needed to do was to 'change our attitude'. Here are some of the things I've seen written about weight management that are supposed to be motivating:

- 'No Excuses.'
- 'Only weak people quit.'
- 'Get your best body ever.'
- 'You can do anything you set your mind to.'
- 'You don't get the arse you want by sitting on it.'
- 'Making excuses burns zero calories per hour.'
- 'Your only limit is you.'
- 'If you're tired of starting over, stop giving up.'
- 'The hard part isn't getting your body in shape. The hard part is getting your mind in shape.'

Apparently, we can just write them down on a piece of paper, put them next to our mirror (or on our fridge) and, low and behold, the weight will drop off! So simple! If you're feeling hopeless about life, I'm sure there's nothing a good quote can't fix after all. I will tell this to my friend Kate, who had both legs amputated at the knee and gained weight due to her medications and, you know, NOT BEING ABLE TO WALK. Dear Kate, you won't get the arse you want by sitting on it... I'm sure she will be inspired to change as a result. It's obviously absurd to say something like that to my friend Kate. What's not so obvious is how absurd these statements are for other people too. And this is because of an issue I have already highlighted—beliefs in a shallow psychological space cannot battle core motivational drivers.

To be fair, there are some beliefs that are actually quite strong. The reality is that not all beliefs are of equal strength. Beliefs that sit in a deep psychological space and consistently impact motivation are called core beliefs. They are beliefs that develop in childhood and remain with us. An example of this might be the belief that 'no one will love me'. There would be a reason that a belief like this develops in childhood—perhaps being abandoned by a parent or experiencing severe bullying. I would anticipate that this influences the development of personality traits and values, which are also deeply embedded in the psyche. A person with this core belief may therefore develop an emotionally unstable personality trait and their values may be strongly drawn to conformity and security. As such, this person can't just come up with a 'new attitude'.

I have witnessed firsthand what happens when we try to get people to change their beliefs and attitudes. There was a trend among mental health clinicians for many years to try and help people with a mental illness 'change their dysfunctional thinking'. Therapists would spend hours exploring beliefs and coming up with evidence to identify these thoughts as being 'wrong'. The aim was for the client to develop new beliefs and to try to embed them in their thinking. But the result was a battle. People were literally battling their own thoughts and therefore battling themselves. It took energy to maintain this battle and people would get tired and then give up. Why? Because battles are psychologically unsustainable. Long-term studies now show these strategies may have a short-term impact, but are difficult to sustain—just like weight loss battles!

We do respond to new information and there has been a significant push in the last few decades to improve people's knowledge and understanding of weight, nutrition and activity levels. But knowledge doesn't always translate into changed behaviour. In fact, health professionals experience higher levels of chronic disease than the general population, and GPs are just as likely to be overweight as the rest of us! If knowledge were enough to motivate people, our health professionals would be healthier. However, having the most knowledge about health doesn't translate into having better health outcomes. Just because people *intend* to behave a certain way doesn't mean that they do. Remember, seventy-five per cent of our behaviour comes from subconscious forces. I intended to have a tidy desk at work after all! New information can be very good at changing our *intentions*, but it is not so helpful at changing our behaviours. And what I can see happening as a result of the disparity between intentions and behaviours is guilt and hopelessness, both poor motivators for sustainable change.

There have been some other unfortunate and unintended outcomes as a result of the push to inform and educate us about weight. Inadvertently, such outcomes have given the community the message that people are to blame for their health issues. This was suggested to my friend Elizabeth when she went to see her GP. But from my experience, weight is often a RESULT of health problems. My administration officer only gained significant weight after going on steroids to treat her asthma. My friend Kate only gained weight after they removed her second leg and changed her medications. My clients in mental health services only gained weight when they were put onto psychiatric medications. I only gained weight while experiencing depression and hopelessness. A colleague only gained weight after experiencing a workplace injury and being bedridden for months. My mother gained weight because of arthritis in her knee. And yet we always assume the reverse is the truth. We assume people are depressed because of their weight, not that their depression caused their weight. We assume knees are sore because of weight gain, not that weight developed as a result of sore knees. But often, people's attempts to manage an injury or condition is the precipitator and not as simple as changing an attitude.

The truth is that the well-intentioned health campaigns have also created a level of arrogance in our community about weight. Instead of looking at the issue in a holistic manner that includes medications, mental health, grief, illness or injury, we jump to conclusions about the person's personality, their priorities or their habits. I know people far larger than myself who exercise more and eat a more healthful diet than I do. So, assumptions are very damaging and very tiresome. I was reading an article recently about a larger woman who was going to the gym regularly. She had been going for years and was in fact quite fit. One of the problems she kept facing was that other people in the gym assumed she was there to lose weight and kept 'encouraging' her by saying things such as 'keep up the good work' and 'you'll get there'. She found this assumption deeply patronising. In reality, she was probably fitter than most of them. Unless you are someone's personal physician, you cannot assume to know anything about an overweight person's health. Just as you do not know anything about a slim person's health.

Health campaigns focused on getting us to change our behaviour to manage our weight have inadvertently started blaming ALL people who gain weight, without a contextual reference. We have literally taken on the 'no excuses' way of thinking. Not only is this inaccurate, but it damages the motivation of people who find themselves in these situations. It has added shame to the equation, and shame is *demotivating.* In all the years I have worked with people and their motivation, I have never seen a single person bring positive change into their lives through shame. Never. Not once. And that's because shame adds to hopelessness. And hopelessness leads to giving in. And giving in leads to the exact behaviour we want to stop. This isn't rocket science, and yet over and over again people try and use shame to *motivate other people*. It is the worst thing anyone can ever do to someone that needs to make a change.

I'm sure many of you heard the story of a young model who took a photo of an older woman naked in the gym shower room. Posting it on social media, her comment with the post was 'If I can't unsee this than neither can you'. We know nothing about this older woman, but let me tell you about the women in their seventies that I know. They have born and raised children, they have cared for grandchildren, they have survived illnesses, bankruptcy, betrayal and the deaths of people they have loved. They have worked and travelled and volunteered and contributed to the world in amazing ways. I am sure the woman who was photographed did all these things too. And yet she was shamed by a woman who the world claims to be beautiful. I don't know the woman in the photograph, but if I ever get the chance to meet her, I want to thank her for taking care of her body and her health in her seventies. I want to thank her for all the amazing things she's done in her seventy years of life. And I want to say the only thing I saw in that image was complete and utter beauty. I saw my mother, my grandmothers, my aunts and my future self.

I don't believe the young model who took the photo was evil. I believe she has lived in a world that somehow led her to believe that body-shaming was not only acceptable, but funny. And we have all contributed in some way to that world. Every time we criticise our own bodies or someone else's body, we contribute to that world. Every time we talk about a 'good' body versus a 'bad' body, we contribute to that world. Every time we hold up only one type of beauty as being acceptable, we contribute to that world. And so, while this young woman needs to be responsible for her actions, we also need to be responsible for ours. We contributed to the world that led her to believe another human being's perfectly acceptable body was somehow repulsive. But the body was not repulsive, it was the belief that was repulsive.

Thankfully the world saw this incident as a wake-up call. Sometimes one shocking incident can move us out of our complacency. If we can take something good out of the situation, it was that the community stood up and said 'no more' to body-shaming. But will we all do our part to create a world where that is truly possible? Or will we just blame the ones who step so far outside the boundaries of acceptability? If we shame our own bodies, don't we shame everyone's? Can we really be outraged by one young woman's actions when we have all shamed bodies to *some* degree, even when those bodies are our own?

I've also known scenarios where people have tried to use fear as a motivator for change when it comes to weight. The 'if you don't do something right now you will die' approach. While the information may be factual, if it is delivered in a manner intended to produce fear, there can be some problematic consequences. Firstly, using fear as a motivator raises dubious ethical concerns. Is deliberately using fear causing more harm than good? This is something debated in the literature on health promotion. The second issue is that fear has an impact on how we process information. This is particularly true when we believe we have little control to change the issue at hand. I discovered research that suggested we develop a bias against information when it causes us fear. It happens at an information-processing level. We interpret the information as being less valid because it scares us. That is, we literally convince ourselves that it can't be true. As a result, we develop strong internal arguments that counteract the information (much like we do when our autonomy is threatened). When I read this, the first thing that came to my mind were the people who do not believe humans have impacted climate change. Are they so scared they are literally unable to process the information? Does that explain some of the seemingly irrational arguments on the topic? `Overall, fear is a difficult thing to use as a motivator. Again, it may actually drive our thinking in the opposite direction.

As a community, we have received a lot of information about weight management and obesity. I feel that most of us are now reasonably well informed. When educated people continue to have information pushed at them, they start to feel nagged.

This triggers off the need for autonomy again. Community-level health campaigns also have a very limited effect on behaviour. The research indicates that only about seven per cent of the population change their behaviour as a result of promotional campaigns. My concern would be what percentage of the population has their autonomy instinct triggered.

Education has a threshold of impact—it can only take people so far. And it is too easily influenced by misinformation. The idea of superfoods is an example of information being exaggerated. While the foods labelled as 'super' all have nutritional value and can be a helpful addition to a diet, to claim anything is super about them really stretches the argument. A colleague of mine recently came to a work celebration with a cacao, chia seed, gluten-free, coconut oil chocolate cake. I would rather eat cake with butter and sugar! We all want to believe in the possibility of superfoods, but the reality is most foods have something 'super' about them. And it is really the variation and diversity of our diets that adds nutrients more so than any one food we consume.

There is of course an irony I must admit to as I write this chapter. I am in fact targeting your beliefs and attitudes to create a positive change. And I suppose that's the thing to consider. New information can be helpful. But as human beings, we are more sophisticated than just 'getting a positive attitude'. We need individualised information that works with who we are and where we are at. Don't get me wrong, I love a good quote. I have used some of my favourites throughout this book! But quotes don't change the world. They add to an already complex mix of motivational drivers and should be used with caution and consideration.

CHAPTER 12

Willpower

> *'Do not let what you can't do, stop you from doing what you can'*
>
> — John Wooden

Willpower is your friend. Have you ever had one of those friends though who promises to come to a party but often doesn't show up? Who forgets your birthday? Who borrows things and never returns them? Who is always late? Who tries hard, but can't be relied upon? That friend is like your willpower—well intentioned but unreliable. Don't expect too much from willpower—it will only disappoint you!

If you understand your willpower and acknowledge its limitations, you can get quite a lot out of it. There's a reason you keep an unreliable friend in your life—when they are there, they are fabulous! It's just that you don't always know when they are going to show up. In fact, using willpower wisely will be one of the keys to weight management across your lifespan. But willpower gets easily distracted and easily led astray. It is influenced by everything and anything—a fleeting thought, a moment of doubt, a headache, a craving, a badly worded email, tiredness or a lapse in concentration. As long as you understand its capacity, you will not be disappointed. But if you think willpower will help you solve major life issues like weight management, you're in for a fall, I'm afraid.

Willpower is the determination to carry out a decision, goal or plan despite challenges or temptations. Willpower gets far too much credit for weight management. The reality is, willpower is something that exists only in a moment in time. Its strength is so variable, it can change moment by moment, day by day. In fact, there is research that shows our ability to use willpower depletes through the day. If you're wondering why you are more likely to binge eat at night, this is your answer! Remember the metaphor of the little girl in a tug of war? The little girl can do fine if all she is doing is pulling against another little girl of the same age and weight. However, if the little girl is pulling against a grown man, she's going to need some extra muscle power on her team to be competitive. The little girl is willpower. The real muscle power comes from your deep motivational drivers.

People have called me 'a dog with a bone' when I really want to get something done. Time and time again, I show endless determination to fight battles, get through struggles and find the patience to push through barriers. I have endless willpower when it comes to some things. All these things sit in my strong values profile for universalism, beneficence and self-direction. I will not do this when it comes to achievement values, face values or conformity values. That was why writing academically was a struggle for me. It wasn't that I lacked willpower, it was that I lacked the strong motivational drivers to support my willpower *for this task*. While I can look like a person who has tremendous willpower, the reality is I only have tremendous willpower when it works on the same team as my strong motivational drivers.

Other people are like this too. Whenever you look at someone else and admire their willpower with something, it is only functioning in that manner because it is built on a team of deep intrinsic drivers. People who never eat cake or ice-cream appear to have really strong willpower when it comes to eating. But they are using willpower in conjunction with deeper forces such as their personality, their passion or their values. The same goes for people who have tidy houses, who study hard, who spend hours volunteering or raising money, who grow their own produce, who live on a tight budget. If people appear to have strong willpower, it is only ever because it fits with something deeper and stronger in their motivational profile. But willpower gets all the credit, and it's time for that fantasy to stop.

Below, I have created diagrams to represent the strength of my motivation for writing this book versus the strength of my motivation for exercise. Overall, motivation is created through a combination of all the drivers working together. I have completed the diagrams by representing the components of motivation as different width bars—the stronger the motivational component, the wider the bar in the diagram.

My motivation for writing this book

Let's look in detail at the motivational drivers we have spoken about so far in this book. The diagram is at the end of the descriptions I have provided.

Passion

Writing is a passion of mine and I define myself as a 'writer'. Therefore, the passion driver is very wide in the diagram.

Values

The topic of this book is strongly allied with my personal values. The aim of my book is to help other people understand themselves better. As a result, the motivational driver related to values is also quite wide.

Hope

Hope is an interesting one for writing this book, because I have never published a book before. As such, I have a lot to learn and am not entirely sure about my skills. Hope is present, but in comparison to the other drivers for writing, it is somewhat narrower.

Autonomy

I am in control of the content of the book and I am able to choose the timeframe for writing the book. As a result, the autonomy driver is reasonably wide.

Personality

Writing connects with my personality for openness and new experiences. As an introvert, I am also happy to spend hours of my time alone with my writing. The personality driver is therefore strong.

Intuition

I have a deep intuition that I should write this book and do it now. It is also helping me with the content as I write. I believe my greater purpose in life is to be a writer. This motivational driver is therefore very powerful.

Beliefs & Attitudes

I have enough knowledge about the topic, which links to attitudes and beliefs. I certainly don't know everything about motivation, but I feel I have enough information to talk about the topic with some degree of insight. As a result, this driver is fairly wide.

Willpower

Am I required to use willpower to write this book? Yes. I have had to spend time reading and researching as the book has emerged. This has required self-discipline. I also set myself a timeline for completing the initial draft, so this has encouraged me to use willpower when I don't really feel like writing.

Motivation for writing

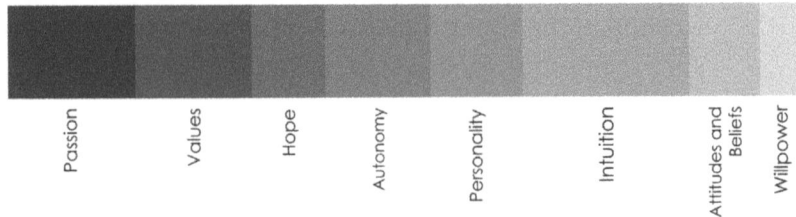

Overall, my motivational profile for writing this book is very strong. I am using willpower, but as you can see from my description, the real power of my motivational forces is coming from other drivers. Willpower is just helping me to focus and get the book completed in a timeframe. It is enhancing my motivation but not giving it any real power.

My motivation for exercise

Now compare this to the motivational drivers I have for exercise.

Passion

Exercise is not a passion of mine. I like it, but it is not something I naturally do when tired or busy. This makes it a narrow motivational force.

Values

I value my health, which links to humility and beneficence. I want to be there for my children and I want to be well enough to fulfil my life purpose. Exercise therefore links reasonably strongly to my values.

Hope

Hope is pretty strong, even compared to my hope for the book. This is because I am currently managing to exercise regularly, four or five times a week. Motivationally this is quite wide.

Autonomy

I am able to choose what exercise I do and when, without any feeling of guilt, which enhances my sense of autonomy. However, there is still some sense of community expectation that feels like it impeded my autonomy to some degree.

Personality

We discovered earlier that my personality profile is not very strong when it comes to exercise. I don't like rigid routines and goals, and have a lower level of self-control because of my low conscientiousness trait. The motivational band is therefore quite narrow.

Intuition

Intuition tells me to exercise, however, it feels slow and encouraging rather than urgent. I know it makes me feel better and I know I am now in a space to be able to accommodate exercise into my life.

Attitudes & Beliefs

My attitudes and beliefs definitely support regular exercise. I know that exercise will help my health in the longer term and I believe it is an activity worth doing regularly.

Willpower

And then there is willpower—small portion at the end of my motivational profile urging me on. It's there when I have that moment of thinking, 'It's been two days since I have done any exercise. I might go for a walk'. It's there when I wake up early and think, 'I have a bit of time this morning. Maybe I should spend fifteen minutes doing yoga.' And it's there when my dog looks at me with pleading eyes that say, 'Please take me for a walk.'

Motivation for exercise

| Passion | Values | Hope | Autonomy | Personality | Intuition | Attitudes and Beliefs | Willpower |

The total width of the diagram for exercise is much narrower than the total width of the diagram for writing. And that demonstrates the strength of motivation for each activity. I am using willpower for writing this book and for exercise. But, willpower is a small component of the overall motivation for both activities.

And willpower sometimes fails in both scenarios.

Willpower is not helpful for writing the book when I have been at work all day and feel tired. Willpower for writing is not helpful when my daughter wants to spend time with me and watch a movie. Willpower is not helpful for writing when the weekend is busy and there are urgent things to get done.

Willpower for exercise is not helpful at five in the morning when I am still sleepy. Willpower for exercise is not helpful when my workday has been long and frustrating and I all I want to do is relax. Willpower for exercise is not present when the weather is rainy or very hot.

So, willpower is there, helping in both scenarios, but it also fails in both scenarios. There are times when I don't 'push through' for either writing or exercise. However, I am more likely to 'push through' for writing because it has a stable base built on strong motivators.

Research talks about willpower as a limited resource. It suggests that any activity that requires considerable self-control leads to a state called 'ego-depletion'. Any time we are required to use self-control, we have less ability to use willpower, again, directly following the activity. There is a limit to what we can do that takes self-control or willpower at any one time. We therefore seek periods of rest following significant use of willpower in order to recoup our resources.

Those of you who have experienced the joys of parenting will know how much self-control it requires. No wonder there is no energy left to resist a muffin at the end of the day! Let me share some of my personal parenting stories that required significant self-control.

- My eighteen-month-old daughter took a grape off the bunch and then decided she wanted it to go back onto the bunch. The fact that the grape wouldn't go back onto the bunch led to an enormous tantrum. I knew at that moment I was in for an interesting journey.

- The first time we experienced head lice in our home was also fun. I had both children in the bath with a lice treatment in their hair. It needed to stay on for half an hour to be effective. Evan did a poo in the bath during this waiting time. I had to get both children out of the bath while they still had the treatment in their hair, remove the poo, clean the bath, and put them back in. I then spent the next hour combing nits out of their hair while they both screamed. Ah, good times!

- Once I heard a loud noise and discovered my son had been playing with cans of soft drink in the living area. One of the cans had exploded, soaking him and leaving soft drink on my ceiling, down my walls, on the floor, lounge and television. I continued to find dried soft drink for at least three months following the incident.

- Another great poo story happened when I was toilet-training my two-year-old daughter. She was happy to pee on the potty but insisted she wanted her nappy back on to poo. After months of this I'd had enough, and one day I refused to put her nappy back on. Obviously, I became the evil mother and so she went in search of Daddy. The next thing I heard was my husband scream my name, so I went upstairs to look for him. At the top of the stairs on my pale cream carpet was an enormous poo that had clearly been stepped in. I found my husband in the bathroom holding our two-year-old over the toilet while hopping on one foot. The other foot was in the air covered in poo. That stain never came out of the carpet despite hours of trying and hundreds of dollars on professional carpet cleaning.

- Another time, my son decided he would play the drums on my timber coffee table with the metal meat tenderiser. There is a reason we no longer buy nice things.

- One day my daughter told me at eight pm that she had an assignment due the next day, which she hadn't' started yet. The assignment was to be on volcanoes. Let's just say I contained an eruption of sorts in our house that night!

- I was outside hanging washing on the line and returned to the house to find my son and the dog sitting on the lounge and sharing an entire roll of expensive brie. They were having the most delightful time! I have also come in from the washing line to find Evan eating mango from the dirty dog bowl. Perhaps I need to stop washing…

These stories are just snippets of normal parenting drama. There are hundreds of stories of frustration and patience and downright despair. Of all the things in life that take self-control, surely parenting is one of the most demanding. If willpower is weak whenever we are required to use a lot of self-control, it is no wonder the advent of parenting also happens to be the advent of weight gain for many of us! Imagine adding on top of normal parenting, a child with a developmental delay and autism, and I think you can see self-control in our house is a daily struggle. I have often told my husband that the children take up ninety-five per cent of my patience, which leaves only five per cent for him and the rest of the world. I now have research to back me up on this statement!

There are many books out there on willpower, and there is even research on how to get the most out of your willpower, but I am not convinced this is time well spent. Our willpower will fluctuate. It is natural for it to work in this manner. We need to rest to rebuild resources when it comes to self-control and this informs me that, if we rely too much on willpower to manage our weight, we will end up depleted. And what happens then? Binge eating is probably the reality. I believe it is better to work with our willpower as a natural, although inconsistent, resource.

Willpower is no place to build our house of weight management strategies. Continuous denial and use of willpower are not going to be effective in a task that goes over a lifetime. I said in the first chapter of this book that I do not battle myself. If willpower is weak, I am okay with that. I simply think, 'I can't do that today'. If willpower is strong, I embrace the moment. Neither of these states is right or wrong. They are what they are on any given day in any given moment. No guilt and no frustration. I expect willpower to change and to fluctuate. I expect it to be powerful at times and weak at others. This is normal human motivation, not dysfunctional willpower. If we can understand willpower for what it is rather than fantasise that it is the source of superior motivation, we can be kinder to ourselves and much more effective at finding strategies that work in the long term. Willpower is simply a helpful although unreliable addition to other motivational drivers you have at your disposal. Willpower is great for having a slightly smaller piece of cheesecake: it will help you exercise when you feel a bit flat or it can assist you in choosing a lower fat pizza topping. But it cannot help you deny yourself day and night for years to come. It was never designed for this purpose.

CHAPTER 13

Goals

'One of the hardest things in life to learn are which bridges to cross and which bridges to burn'

— Oprah Winfrey

I have had many goals in life that I didn't achieve. The book you are reading isn't the first book I've attempted to write. I started writing a book after becoming a mother and finding myself in a world that felt overwhelming. I abandoned that book once I realised I had bigger problems on my hands, with a child that was not developing as expected. I also had a goal that I would be a wonderful gardener. I had bursts of enthusiasm over several years where I would buy lots of plants only to discover the green thumb I thought I wanted took more effort than I was prepared to give. The number of poor, dead plants I have found in my garden is not something that gives me pride. I had a goal to live a more environmentally sustainable life and ditch my love of plastic wrap. This unfortunately ended the first day I couldn't find a clean container for my son's school sandwich. There are so many things I *want* to be. And there are so many things I am not.

I think we all have this fantasy of being 'better'. My mother is in her sixties and retired from being a schoolteacher. She's told me that she thought once she retired she would 'finally get organised'. To her dismay, retirement did not come with a magic organisational wand. She was not happy when I laughed at her and told her if she wasn't organised by now, she never would be. The aim of constantly improving is an admirable one, but it is often not our reality. Some people say the greatest predictor of future behaviour is past behaviour after all.

There are many advocates for setting a good goal. Over and over again, you will hear people talk about the positive impact of goal setting and how, without a goal, you only have a dream. There are many places in life where goals have great value. Planning a vacation, completing a degree, buying a car, starting a charitable foundation—these are all great goals to have. But losing weight and keeping it off? This is where I struggle with the idea of goal setting.

Weight management is a practice, not a goal. A goal suggests an end point, it suggests an achievement, and it suggests something you can tick off a list. Just like the examples I gave above. They all have an end point. But when it comes to weight management, there is no end point. Managing weight is something that requires daily focus. It's like brushing our teeth, having a shower or washing our clothes. It has to be done daily for the rest of our lives. You can't 'do' weight management and tick it off the list.

There is considerable research about the effectiveness of goals. I am not disputing the research that exists. I am suggesting that a specific goal related to long-term daily practice may not be the *most effective* approach. It's about longevity, not achievement. There are many practices that have an impact on health—deep breathing, spending time in nature, laughter, good quality friendships, marriage, music, gratitude, spirituality, optimism (oh, and let's not forget knitting). We don't usually set goals around these things. They naturally exist in our day-to-day lives. We are already motivationally inclined towards them. And to me, weight management needs to be more like this type of behaviour and less like a goal.

After reading so much about motivation, I would also speculate that the process of goal setting doesn't suit everyone's 'style'. The conscientious personalities probably love a good goal. I can imagine they thrive under the structure of it. But what about the people with less conscientious personality traits? Perhaps the people who strongly value achievement work well with goals. They would love the idea of challenging themselves to complete a difficult task. But this synchronicity may only work with some motivational profiles.

It seems an assumption exists that when we set a goal, carrying out the tasks leading to the goal will eventually lead to a habit. I found no evidence for this in the research. We think a goal such as 'I will go to the gym three times a week' will just become a part of everyday life. I discuss habits in chapter fourteen and it does not seem as simple as we'd like to believe.

Goal setting is likely to be similar to willpower in that the deeper layers of our motivation may be the true influence rather than the goal setting process per se. I set a goal to write this book, for example, but the reason I set that goal is that it connects with my core motivational drivers. A goal might add or enhance the overall process, but it is not the motivational force behind the activity. The reason I set a goal to write this book was to have a draft ready by a certain date, not because I wasn't motivated to achieve the goal. I have not procrastinated, and I have not felt 'unmotivated' about writing this book. That is because it is so deeply embedded within my core drivers. Goal setting is not useless in this scenario, but it is also not the reason I am achieving what I want to do. Goal setting simply organises my motivation, it doesn't create it.

It's not that goals are bad. It's just that strong goals need to be set on a foundation of strong motivational drivers. As such, I believe they would be far more achievable. My herb garden kept dying because I wanted a garden, but I wasn't a gardener. The *why* of the goal is therefore probably more important than the process of actually setting the goal. I would still be motivated to complete this book without a specific and measurable goal in place. In fact, I can barely *stop* myself from writing this book! And that's what people look like when they are motivated from their core drivers—focused and determined, not tortured and exhausted.

I noticed this in my practice as a mental health clinician several years ago. Health services kept setting goals, but the reasons behind many of the goals were not strong enough to *drive people*. My colleagues would often 'start small' when helping people with goals. They would recommend something that seemed simple and easy to achieve. Activities such as 'going to the supermarket' were often a starting point. Their philosophy was that this would give people a sense of achievement, a boost in confidence, and then they could build on it with more complex and challenging goals. And while logical, this was often not what happened. Many people seemed to get stuck at the starting goal. As health services, we weren't harnessing the real power of motivation that existed within our clients. This only occurred when we linked into the deeper layers of their motivation. People would push through all types of barriers—anxiety, fear, a lack of confidence, the need to learn new skills—for the things they *really* cared about. People could manage all types of challenges if the motivation came from a deep source. But they would do none of these things for goals that sat in a shallower motivational space. I learnt this directly from the people I saw with sparks of energy, not from a book or a model. I simply asked myself the question, 'What made that person so energised and excited about *this* particular goal?'

However, it was hard to find tools that would assist me to have conversations with my clients about these 'deeper motivators'. As a result, I developed my own. The tool is a set of cards called 'Interest Cards'. Each card has a different interest or passion on it and I then get people to sort through the cards and place each interest in a pile of three: strong interests; moderate interests; no interest. This then forms the basis of a much more sophisticated conversation where we can explore the things that provide the most motivational force. It also clearly identifies the areas that will not motivate people. These are the types of conversations we need to start having with people if we really want to find the 'spark' beneath the lack of motivation.

There's another key point I'd like to make about the topic of goals that doesn't seem to be well documented. You see, the research is all about achieving the goal. And yes, people who have a goal are more likely to achieve that goal. But what happens after that goal is achieved? What happens a year, two years or five years after the goal has been achieved?

There is a concept called 'hedonic adaptation'. Research demonstrates that people 'adapt' to things that make them happy. When this thing that brought happiness becomes the 'norm', it no longer brings them happiness. While I haven't seen these concepts linked, I would speculate there's a physiological reason related to dopamine that drives this response. Dopamine is that feel-good neurotransmitter that acts as a chemical reward system. When we achieve our goals, we get a rush of dopamine and we feel happy. But as time goes on, and we get used to what we have achieved, it would be logical to conclude we no longer experience as many dopamine peaks. We therefore go back to being as happy as we were before we achieved the goal. This process happens quite quickly, usually within the space of a year.

The good news is the same system works when something bad happens as well. At first, we are upset and unhappy, but, after a while, we go back to being about as happy as we were before the bad thing happened. Things that seem awful, such as paraplegia, don't make people as unhappy as we might assume. At least not in the long term. The process of adapting to something bad can take longer than the adaptation to happiness. Eventually though, we adjust to our new circumstances and move forward with as much happiness or misery as we had before!

Hedonic adaptation is the reason why winning the lottery doesn't make you happier. Winners eventually go back to being their old grumpy selves! The same thing happens with other major life goals—buying a house, getting married, going on a holiday, receiving a promotion, finishing university or buying a new car. We strive and strive and strive for our goal, and it makes us temporarily happy. And then what do we do? We set a new goal. We are never actually content with where we are at. And this is one of the problems with goal setting. We can goal-set our entire lives and never actually be happy. We just get temporary hits of dopamine.

I will take an educated guess that this is also what happens when people diet and hit their target weight. They initially feel great and it does in fact make them happy. But this is a temporary feeling. Let's imagine Connie sets a goal to lose ten kilograms. She decides to take a sensible approach and searches for a weight loss program that focuses on good quality food and exercise. She finds a program where she gets to set her own menu plans and loves what she sees. There are people on the website she can relate to, people who look like mothers and grandmothers. No one seems to be showing off in a bikini. She sets the goal of losing the weight within four months. This seems like a very sensible and realistic goal. She starts the program with great enthusiasm and almost immediately she sees results by losing 1.5 kilograms in the first week. This gives her a rush of dopamine and she becomes even more enthusiastic than she was before. Connie keeps to the program with only a few 'lapses' and hits her target weight within her designated timeframe.

Connie feels this has been a real achievement. She has gone down a clothing size and people keep commenting on how great she looks—dopamine, dopamine, dopamine. Eventually people stop commenting and Connie becomes used to her new shape. She no longer feels quite so excited when she buys clothes a size smaller. She is still proud of what she has achieved, but it's not quite so exciting. The sense of reward is now a thought as opposed to a physiological release of dopamine. In fact, it starts to become the new norm. She still has all the same problems she had before she lost the weight—her son is still struggling at school, her husband is still stressed at work, her mother still complains about everything and the bills are still hard to pay on time. Without the strong sense of achievement and release of dopamine, the weight she lost is a little less satisfying. She starts to slip and realises she has gained two kilograms. How did that happen so quickly? She feels angry with herself. Dopamine is no longer in high supply. Instead, she has a release of cortisol from the stress she experiences. She punishes herself with more exercise. Rather than feeling positive and excited about what she is doing, she feels desperate to 'get it under control'. These negative feelings start to impact hope. And you know where the story goes from there.

This is a motivational pattern I suspect happens when people have a set goal for weight management. At first it can lead to a sense of success and help to keep people motivated. Dopamine is helping sustain motivation because it is giving a feeling of pleasure. But the long-term impact of goal setting is less clear, and certainly we know people who 'diet' (i.e. set a clear and specific goal to lose weight) gain more weight over their lifespan than people who never diet. So, to me, it is not the goal setting we should be examining, it is what happens after the goal has been achieved. Does reaching a goal and then losing it or going backwards make things worse? Do we go from a motivational high to a motivational low? Does it impact hope?

I have lived in a world of goal setting. Healthcare puts a big focus on it and encourages goals in our documentation. Here's the dilemma for me though: I see no evidence that goal setting works in the real world of healthcare. And believe me, I have looked for it. Goals have their place. But is health a destination? Is it something that can be broken down into small, achievable, measurable steps? And once 'achieved', how does one stay there? I think this is where the real problem occurs. Health will fluctuate throughout a person's life. Weight will fluctuate throughout a person's life. And motivation isn't as simple as just setting a goal.

I could have set a specific and measurable goal to write and publish an academic article. I could have persevered and developed the skills required to achieve the goal. I could have kept to a tight plan and completed the task. It would have made me successful when it came to the goal. What it wouldn't have made me successful at was living authentically and listening to my intuition. My goal success would have in fact been a life failure. I needed to go partially down that path to realise it was wrong for me. I needed to feel the struggle with my motivation to identify that it was not the right path. I am deeply, deeply grateful I did not achieve that goal. It could have taken me on a journey to misery—being successful at goals but not successful in my life. I probably wouldn't have written this book if I had achieved it. Sometimes the most successful thing you can do is abandon a goal!

If weight management is a practice and not a goal, it needs to be able to adapt and change to all the ups and downs of life. It needs to be an act of kindness and love to oneself, not an act of punishment. And I don't see rigid goals as being helpful in a space that needs this much flexibility. Goals are designed to be inflexible. That's how they work. You are supposed to 'push through' challenges and obstacles, like a bulldozer. But what if we thought about health more like it was an ocean, a moving and changing thing that accommodated the challenges of life? Something that moved with and around obstacles rather than tried to push through them?

I believe we are motivationally better off having a weight range we aim to stay within—a space of four or five kilograms that accommodates holidays and illness and busy work schedules and changes in caring responsibilities. I have personally found this a better option for myself. I aim to exercise regularly. But when it doesn't happen, I have not failed. I aim to eat as many vegetables as I can. Some days this is easy and, on other days, impossible. I aim to have many other health-enhancing elements in my life: fun, purpose, passion and friends. Health is a multidimensional concept and, at times, aspects of it are going to be harder or easier than others. Rather than fighting against this, we could just accept it as being part of the lifelong process of health. There may be periods where we can and periods where we can't. Acceptance and movement through these periods seems healthier than guilt, pressure and self-loathing.

Goals are great for many things in life—saving to buy a house, completing a renovation, learning to speak another language or trekking up Mount Kilimanjaro. But we need an end point; otherwise, goals may just be another pathway for us to feel like failures.

CHAPTER 14

Habits

'Nothing so needs reforming as other people's habits'

— Mark Twain

My dog Coco can't read, and as far as I am aware she can't understand most of what I say. She certainly can't tell the time and she doesn't know days have names such as Monday or Sunday. But every Saturday morning at seven am she starts scratching at my bedroom door. Once I have arisen, she will follow me around religiously until she sees me get out a certain pair of shoes. At this point she starts barking, jumping and spinning in circles with excitement. Coco knows we are about to go for a walk. Despite not knowing Monday from Sunday, Coco knows exactly what is meant to happen every day of the week and when. She knows when she gets fed, when people are due home, when she is being left at home and when she gets to come along too. She knows certain shoes mean certain things, and that suitcases are a cause for sadness and sulking. She reads this family like a book. Coco is aware of all our habits and all the cues that go with them.

How does she know the difference between Friday and Saturday? Our habits change. How does she know sneakers mean a walk? They are a cue she recognises. You only need to own a dog to know how much we function from habits. Habits are an important functional process. They increase our efficiency and reduce the need for intentional thought. Think about the first five things you do when you get to work each day. I'm pretty sure you can list them easily. Here's my list:

1. Say hello to everyone
2. Put my lunch in the refrigerator
3. Turn my computer on
4. Make a cup of tea
5. Open my email and diary

Every day. Habits are comforting, organising and functional. My administration officer knows not to try and have a conversation with me until I've made my cup of tea. It is disorienting and confusing if she tries!

What are habits? Many people believe habits are an activity or behaviour that we do frequently. That is not quite correct. A real habit only occurs in a particular context with a cue. Coco is using the cue of a pair of shoes to know if I am going to implement my habit of a Saturday morning walk. A cue is something environmental that lets us know something is happening. It can be something we see, hear, smell, touch or taste. Coco can hear our car pulling into our driveway. It cues her that we are about to come home and she then comes to the gate to greet us. Coco knows that she gets fed after we have eaten dinner. When she sees we have finished eating, she makes a fuss about getting fed. Coco knows that, when we turn off the lights, it is time for bed. She gets herself into her sleeping position as we turn off the lights. The cue is the lights going off and the habit is going to bed.

We use cues all the time. The purpose of a cue is to reduce the amount of thinking and problem-solving we have to do. It is efficient for our brains to use cues. When we hear an alarm, we stop and look for danger. We don't think, 'What is that noise and why is it so loud?' An alarm has been set in our minds to have a particular sound and a particular meaning. It is a socially constructed cue for danger. When we greet someone and they hold out their hand, we reach out to shake it. This obviously is a cue for us to engage in a handshake. When we go to a lecture, we become quiet when we see the lecturer stand at the front and look around the room. It is a cue they are about to start speaking. So, cues are very helpful in assisting us to solve problems and be efficient with our mental energy. Once we know the cue, we don't have to spend time thinking about what is required. And cues also help us to develop habits.

Habits are behaviours that happen frequently and use a particular cue in a particular context to trigger them. Habits can be weak or they can be strong. Strong habits are harder to break than weak ones (no surprises there). The degree of repetition and the duration of the behaviour at least partially explains why some habits are weak and why some are strong, although I will argue in this chapter that other factors may also play a role.

Habits account for about forty-five per cent of our daily behaviours (van't Riet, 2011). This is a considerable influence. We know habits influence everything from our snacking to our grocery shopping. The fact that they are also automatic in nature should mean that a change in habits can have an enormous influence on weight management. In fact, health information often targets habits in the way they discuss bringing about positive change. And it sounds really simple and really logical. If you start something new you want to embed as a habit, you are on your way to success with weight management! But like a lot of things relating to motivation and weight management, the simplicity if this idea doesn't quite add up to what we see in real life. Surely if it were this simple, we'd all be doing it by now.

One myth we need to bust is the idea that it only takes twenty-one days to form a new habit. There is no research supporting this simple notion. I know, because I looked for it. What does exist is a study by Philippa Lally and colleagues that demonstrated it could take anywhere from 18 to 254 days to create a habit, and that the average time in the study was in fact 66 days. The first point to take on board is that habit development is extremely VARIABLE. What is mind-blowing about this study is that fifty per cent of the research subjects dropped out and were not included in the analyses because they DID NOT FORM A HABIT AT ALL. The subjects were self-selected and chose a behaviour they wanted to form as a healthy habit. But fifty per cent were unable to even get to the habit-forming stage. To me, this says a lot about just how complex habit development can be. It is not as simple as just doing something on a regular basis.

While I love research and have spent many hours poring over it, there are limitations to the way research is done. Research inevitably takes very small components of motivation and attempts to measure aspects of that component. For example, the research on willpower, habits, autonomy, values, personality, etc. were all completed in separate studies by different groups of researchers. In fact, many of the researchers have spent their entire careers researching just one component of motivation. But that's not how people work. People and their motivation function from a combination of all these elements. You'll find research and books that just focus on the topic of 'habits' or the topic of 'willpower', and yet often the whole picture remains a mystery. Habits cannot be removed from values or from personality when it comes to motivation, but that is not how research is conducted.

Habits can be strong or weak in nature. But why? Are strong habits the ones that correlate with the person's values profile? Are they ones that work in combination with passions or personality? Habits do not function in a vacuum from other motivational drivers. Inevitably we end up in another scenario in which some habits may be easier to develop than others. Some habits may be easier to break than others.

Let me ask you some questions…

What do you drink when you eat pizza?

What do you eat when you go to the cinema?

What do you consume when you meet up with your best friend?

I can guarantee you have habits for all these things. I drink cola when I eat pizza; the only time I eat popcorn is at the cinema;

and my favourite thing to have with my friend Emma is a cup of tea (or maybe three). Emma gave tea up for a period and I nearly lost my mind. It was our ritual! It was what we did together. We'd sit, talk and have cup of tea after cup of tea. I actually felt grief when she stopped drinking it. Inevitably, things that are habits also have meaning. I wanted to be a supportive friend. Emma gave up tea because she liked to have sugar in it. She found it easier to have no tea than to have tea without sugar. I accepted her decision to quit tea, and yet I really struggled with the change because it held such a deep meaning to me. It had a value that went beyond just a habitual behaviour. It would have been easy to sabotage her new 'no tea' goal as a result, and I think this happens frequently when people are trying to make a change.

I have watched many people go through the process of trying to give up smoking. One of the things that amazed me was how other smokers attempted to sabotage a smoker trying to quit. It took me a long time to realise it was because it had a meaning to the other smokers. Think about it. Smokers at work will often have breaks at the same time and go out together to have a cigarette. The habit is not only the act of smoking, it is the act of connecting with friends over smoking. People can form deep relationships while smoking. And they miss their smoking friend as I missed my tea-drinking friend. So, it became more than a habit—tea drinking with my friend became a ritual. Something with meaning. And this then created a loss, not just for Emma, the person attempting to change the habit, but for other people involved in the activity.

I had a colleague who had an annual quit-smoking ritual. She would stop smoking in the middle of the year and work really hard. She usually gained a couple of kilograms in the process. It would take months of effort for her to stop and then she'd try to lose the extra weight. Every year, at Christmas, she started smoking again. On more than one occasion, I watched other smokers entice her back to it. She was often under the influence of a wine or two and another smoker would offer her a cigarette. All that hard work seemed to disappear from her memory and she would accept one. If she accepted one, she inevitably accepted more. On one such occasion, I begged the smoker not to give her a cigarette. They just smiled at me and handed her one. I couldn't comprehend their flippant reaction at the time, but I now understand there's nothing a smoker loves more than someone coming back to the smoking fold.

I personally hate it when people refer to alcohol as 'empty calories'. They of course are referring to the fact that alcohol has no nutritional value. But let me tell you why I can't comprehend this reference to alcohol. When I get home from work, I have a habit of pouring myself a glass of wine. This habit started years ago when my children were toddlers. The late afternoon/evening with small children is usually rather hellish. They are tired, cranky, hungry and sick of following rules. It is the time of day in which major meltdowns are common. They don't want to eat the fish you made them for dinner, despite having told you ten minutes ago they wanted it. They are unhappy with 'that green stuff' you have put onto their plates, and, oh my god, is the mashed potato touching the carrots! Where did their favourite Cinderella drinking cup go to? No, they cannot possibly use the fairy drinking cup even though it is also very pretty. They want to wear their favourite Dora pyjamas, which happen to be in the wash. It seems this time of day brings tears, after tantrum, after torturous and illogical conversation. And, so, Mummy started drinking wine. I would jokingly call it 'happy hour' and tell them there was to be no whingeing, no whining and no crying. In reality, what that small glass of wine meant to me was one slightly indulgent adult moment in the otherwise tantrum-throwing, world-ending chaos that was occurring around me. I would take a sip and remember that life still had some small pleasures among the chaos. And so, a habit formed.

Now that the children are older, things have changed for me during the late afternoon/evening. The moment I walk in the door I get asked 'What are we having for dinner?' despite the fact that it is clearly written on the meal plan posted on the fridge. When I answer, there is inevitable pre-teen eye-rolling, followed by 'Why can't we have takeaway?' When denied, there is stomping to the bedroom until being called down for the apparently terrible food I serve. And so, I still like my glass of wine! I spend ten minutes with my wine, sitting on the balcony enjoying the view before getting up and starting a dinner that no one wants to eat. To call my wine 'empty calories' completely and utterly misses the point. There is nothing empty about this ritual for me. It is still a little bit of grown-up, indulgent pleasure in a chaotic and often frustrating day.

However, if I were to go to a weight loss program, my precious glass of wine would be the first thing a consultant would highlight. They may even use the term 'empty calories'. And superficially, it would seem like the easiest thing for me to give up in order to lose weight. After all, it is a 'bad' habit. But there is one important detail they would be missing: it means a lot to me. Don't get me wrong, as I have gained weight, I have tried to cut back on my wine consumption. I swapped it to a different, low-calorie drink, which worked for about two days. I emptied the house of wine, which lasted a few days more. But I just *missed* it. I truly and genuinely missed that moment of indulgence. It's like my mind suddenly slows and stops thinking about the next thing I have to do. And so, to un-do this apparently 'bad' habit would be extremely difficult. I'm not sure losing weight is enough of a pleasure in comparison to my glass of pinot grigio. When research says that there are strong habits and there are weak habits, I would speculate the meaning behind the habit is one of the main reasons.

I probably have some unhealthy habits though that mean less to me than my evening glass of wine. They may be the habits that could be more easily broken. Another habit is to eat something sweet after my dinner, often a small piece of chocolate. This may be something I could live without. Having read the research about habits and, in particular, how to break bad habits, there was something in the information that concerned me. To break a habit, the recommendation was to change the cue. The cue for my chocolate habit is finishing dinner. How am I supposed to change that cue? Because the habit was a lot weaker though, I thought I would just try and use willpower to make the change. After a couple of weeks, I no longer automatically seek out a piece of chocolate. I found this an interesting experiment.

Upon further exploration, I found another piece of information that might be helpful in breaking habits. The researchers called it 'implementation intentions'. but really, what they mean is make sure you have a clear plan. For my chocolate-eating habit, that would require having an alternative option for the period I would usually eat it. It could include having a piece of fruit to replace the chocolate, because fruit is sweet too. It might involve having a cup of herbal tea instead. Or I have heard of people who clean their teeth straight after a meal to discourage them from eating anything else in the evening. All these things would potentially break the habit.

What about developing new habits? The study I mentioned previously did highlight some useful tips in habit development. The more complex the activity, the harder it was to embed as a habit. They found activities such as 'going for a run' were harder to develop into habits than simpler activities such as 'drink a glass of water'. The other interesting information was that habit formation was easier during the workday than on weekends or holidays. A different study demonstrated that when people are under high stress, they revert to habitual behaviours. The rationale for this finding was that when people are under stress, they want to be as efficient in their thinking as possible and as a result go to the automaticity of habits to function through the challenging time. I believe I relied heavily on habits to get me through my period of hopelessness. There was no way I could have attempted to break an unwanted habit when I was in that space. Perhaps successful habit elimination is as much about timing as anything else.

Habits have some real credibility when it comes to helping people with their health, but we need to know more about how habits work in relationship with other motivational drivers before we have real answers. The benefits of habits are that they are automatic and, once set, are quite easy motivationally to sustain. The problem is getting to that point. Like many things related to motivation, it isn't as simple as making a decision and trying to stick to it.

Section 4

A new perspective

CHAPTER 15

Creating a new relationship with your motivation

'No longer lend your strength to that which you wish to be free from'

— Jewell

Human motivation is an extremely complex issue. It is an individualised process and what works for one person motivationally will not work for someone else. It is therefore ridiculous to take someone else's motivational plan and try to implement it yourself. You are a unique person with a unique motivational profile. Your motivation is not deficient; however, you may be asking things from it that it cannot give you.

The first step in the process is getting to know the motivation you have rather than the motivation you hoped you had. This may take some time, as we have been trained to believe we have a lot of control over our motivation. As you can see from the discussion in the book though, many elements of our motivation are beyond our control. This means we must accept our motivation and find a way to work with it. Pay attention to your motivation without any form of judgement and notice how it works:

- What do you feel most motivationally drawn to?
- What excites you and inspires you?
- What are the things you have tried to battle?
- When does your willpower work?
- When is willpower ineffective?
- What are your values?
- What type of personality do you have?
- What happens with your motivation in the morning?
- What happens in the evening?
- When is activity naturally occurring and enjoyable?
- When is it a struggle?

Your motivation is telling you a story, and it is a story of who you are at your core. These are your strongest and most consistent motivators. If you take the time to listen, without judgement, you will discover the answers to more than just your weight management problems. You will discover yourself as you are designed to be. You will also realise the sales pitch the world has given about who you 'should' be. That person doesn't exist. It is a fairytale as fictional as Cinderella. Our purpose in the world is not perfection. Our purpose is growth. And we cannot grow if we are perfect. It was never part of the design.

I am a writer. I am a giver. I am a food lover. I am a terrible housekeeper. I am an inconsistent exerciser. I am stubborn. I am determined. I am creative. I am generous. I am distractible. I am emotional. I am impatient. I am reflective. I am empathic. I am I. Exactly who I am meant to be. And my motivation is perfect for me and the life I am meant to live.

What my motivation is not perfect for is a world with too much easy access to food and too little movement. It is not perfect for a busy and demanding schedule of competing priorities. It is not perfect for keeping a tidy desk or setting goals. It is not perfect for a size eight pair of jeans. And yet it is my motivational profile that has given me so much. It has taken me on adventures. It has led me to jobs I have loved. It has inspired others. It has generated amazing friendships. It has given me writing and teaching and reflection. It has made me question and explore. It has helped me to be a better mother, a better wife, a better citizen of the world. It has enabled me to grow and to learn. I would choose my motivation again in a heartbeat. Because to want different motivation is to want to be someone else.

If you can accept that your motivation *is* an essential part of your uniqueness, then you can start to have a completely different relationship with it. It gives you the amazing things in your life, as well as the things that frustrate you. The things you *have* achieved have been accomplished because of your motivational profile. The things that have brought you joy and purpose and fulfilment. Your motivation was designed for you so that you could be you. Don't fight it. Don't criticise it. Just understand it, accept it and appreciate it. This is the core message of the book—you are who you are, and your motivation is a very important and powerful part of your individuality.

Do we want to live in a world without givers? Do we want to live in a world where everyone matches their clothes pegs? Do we want to live in a world in which people are only passionate about fitness and nutrition? What would happen to the art and the music and the charities if we lived in that world? Who would make us laugh, make us cry, help us to grow? That's not a world I want.

I am not saying we have no responsibility for taking care of our health. Grown-ups have many responsibilities, and one of them is our health. So, weight management needs to be a focus of our attention and it will take some effort. But it shouldn't be a daily, overwhelming, despairing battle. We have to eat vegetables and we have to be active. But if it requires every bit of effort and energy for us to manage our weight, motivationally that is too much to ask. Because we are not responsible for marketing strategies. We are not responsible for working conditions. We are not responsible for smartphones, computers, cars, televisions, washing machines or any other piece of technology that has made life easier but more sedentary. We are not responsible for our genetics or our dopamine receptors or our cortisol reactivity. There is a balance that needs to be achieved between accepting our biology, utilising the motivation we have and creating an environment in which health and weight management is not such an overwhelmingly difficult task.

The level of responsibility given to individuals needs to be reasonable. It also needs to accommodate personal differences. I can't comprehend a system where we aim for everyone to fit into a particular weight range. Some people have drawn the short straw when it comes to weight management from both biological and motivational components. The last thing they need is to be told their entire lives they are 'overweight'. These people could lose ten per cent of their body mass and still be in a category considered unhealthy. While it may make sense to the health community, motivationally it is not helpful at all.

Take a moment to reflect on your motivation and its strengths. We spend so much time berating our motivation that, instead, let's consider what our motivation has enabled us to do. Everything that is a weakness in one context is a strength in another. The motivation you see as a weakness for weight management has also been a strength for you in other circumstances.

- What are the things your motivation has given you?

- What have you achieved because your motivation took you there?

- Where have you been, who have you loved, what have you given to the world because of your motivation?

If your motivation is an aspect of your uniqueness, have you spent any time being grateful for it? Have you considered what your life would look life if you had a different profile? Would you have different friends, different experiences and different achievements? Who would miss the things you bring to the world right now? To want different motivation is to want to be someone else, and it's quite possible that person isn't as interesting, kind, funny, generous or as happy as you.

If you are not a bikini model, why do you want to look like a bikini model? Seriously. How would your life be better as a result of having a bikini model body? It may be easier to buy clothes, people may admire you more often and you might get more attention, but what else? How many hours of your life are lived needing to wear a swimsuit? Now think about the effort required to have that body against the benefits. Are you prepared to exercise hours a day? Are you prepared to monitor everything that goes into your mouth? Are you prepared to never eat pasta, never drink wine and never have cake? Are you prepared to feel hungry a lot of the time? Are you happy to spend all your energy focused on your shape, your weight, your muscle tone? Are you really, truly prepared to do this for the benefits you would gain?

No? For most of us the benefits are not worth the effort. Which is exactly why we don't do it. Think about what you would have to STOP doing to accommodate a bikini body into your life? Time with your children? Time at work? Time to cook? Time to read? Time to relax? Time with your aging parents or grandparents? Time with friends? Any change requires you to give up something. And if what you need to give up is more important to you, then it will not happen.

My body does everything I need it to. I haven't worn a bikini in at least twenty years. It has not impacted my happiness or my life purpose in any way. I can think, I can see, I can smile, I can type, I can hug, I can talk, I can walk, I can eat, I can pee, I can poop, I can smell, I can laugh, I can cry, I can dance, I can make love. My body is not in pain. My body is not ill. My body is fine. What about yours? If you are like me, why do you need anything different from your body than it is already giving you? Of course, the answer may be no. There may be changes that need to happen so your body can do what it needs. But there is a big difference between a body that does what it needs to and a bikini body. A bikini body is of little use to most of us. Don't envy that body. Instead aim for the body that works for your actual life. Be happy in that body and be grateful for it.

The quote at the start of this chapter states '*No longer lend your strength to that which you wish to be free from*'. Every time we envy someone else's body, we lend strength to the idea that skinny is better. Every time we comment on someone else's weight, we lend strength to the idea that there is something wrong with a body type. Every time we feel bad because we ate a piece of cake, we lend strength to the idea that food is 'good or bad'. Every time we edit our photos, we lend strength to the idea that there is something wrong with us as we are. Every time we complain about our lack of motivation, we lend strength to the idea that our motivation is flawed. If we are sick of these things, we can choose to no longer lend our strength to them.

Don't buy magazines that say someone is pregnant every time they have a slight bump on their abdomen. Don't buy from sellers that refuse to accommodate people of varying sizes. Don't join conversations in which fat people are belittled. Don't share memes that blame people for their health problems. Don't call models that are smaller than the average person 'plus-sized'. Don't wear underwear designed to suck everything in. Our energy is better spent on other, more worthy things. We don't need to feed the beast that enslaves us.

If we don't want to live in a world that idolises thinness, then let's no longer lend *our* strength to it. We are in the *habit* of believing thin is better. We are in the *habit* of believing thin is more attractive. We are in the *habit* of believing thin is healthier. If we really want to break a bad habit, that is the one to focus on. Once we have stopped giving our energy to this delusion, we can focus in a meaningful way on our health. But every time we dishonour our own body and envy someone else's, we add to the strength of the very thing we despise. We have a lot of power. If we started being genuinely grateful for the body we had, would we care for our bodies rather than punish them? Would we nourish our bodies rather than starve them? Would we joyfully move rather than force ourselves to exercise? Would we sleep more, laugh more, love more? These messages would have no power if we all stopped. And we would all be healthier as a result.

These messages damage our motivation for weight management and for genuine health. It's time to stop admiring these people and realise they don't have anything we need. Let's start admiring people who really deserve it. You know what I admire? A mother taking three young children to the supermarket all by herself! That woman is a hero in my opinion. Or someone who is taking in abandoned animals and rehousing them. That's pretty awesome. Or perhaps scientists finding a cure for cancer? Let's admire them instead. There are a million people doing a million things more worthy of our admiration than thinness. And deep down we know that, but we get distracted.

I recently watched a documentary on the Roosevelts and was so enamoured by Eleanor I couldn't stop talking about her. That woman kicked arse! The things she did were amazing. She took on poverty, she took on sexism, she took on racism and she took on social justice. She led the development of the Universal Declaration of Human Rights for goodness sake! And yet she was not pretty, she was not glamourous and she was not thin. But that woman made the world a better place. And maybe she was able to do those things because she wasn't the prettiest girl. The fact that she didn't get distracted by the mirror may have helped her focus her attention on other people and other issues. Her weight never stopped her from doing a damn thing she was supposed to do with her life.

It's time to separate the message of health from the message of weight. It is just one factor in a truly health-focused life. Weight seemed like it would be an easy thing to change. It wasn't. And unless our communities are prepared to consider some radical changes to how our society works, it won't be. Let's focus on an authentic sense of wellness and health rather than a socially constructed one. Does our body feel rested? Do we feel nourished? Do we feel connected to other people? Do we feel purposeful in our lives? Do we feel content? Joyful? Energised? These questions are far more helpful in recognising health than our weight. This is where we need to head if we genuinely want to address the obesity epidemic—a holistic and sustainable definition of health that motivates and encourages people to be exactly who they are meant to be.

CHAPTER 16

Working with the motivation you have

---

*'The great enemy of the truth is very
often not the lie,
deliberate, contrived and dishonest,
but the myth, persistent, pervasive
and unrealistic'*

— John F. Kennedy

We've all been asking the wrong question when it comes to motivation. The question isn't 'How do I get motivated?' The question is 'What motivation do I have?' The idea that we can generate motivation is a myth, one that has been pervasively ingrained into our psyche. The fact that we have all believed it for so long makes it harder to dispute. It's not an easy truth to absorb. And it may require a completely different approach to the issue of obesity than we have been relying upon, but I think it is time we recognised the current approach just hasn't been working. It's not working because it hasn't accommodated the sophistication of human behaviour and the motivation that drives it.

It's time to bust some myths:

- **Fat people are not lazy.**

    They usually feel hopeless, which is a valid and pervasive psychological state.

- **We don't choose our priorities.**

    Our priorities are embedded into our values, which developed in our childhood.

- **Thin people do not have better willpower.**

    They have different core drivers and that is what really enables their behaviour for weight management.

- **The strategies fit, skinny people use to motivate themselves do not work for the rest of us.**

    We are different from them psychologically and this will not change no matter how many goals and plans we put in place.

- **Being fat is not a problem generated by dysfunctional human beings, it is a problem generated by an environment that human beings were never motivationally designed to live in.** The real solutions therefore lie within environmental changes.

The people who have been keeping these myths alive do not have poor intentions, they have poor knowledge. We have not been 'lied' to, we have simply been living under the myth that weight management is simple. It isn't. To continue living under this myth puts us in a dire position. We must work with human beings in a manner that acknowledges how they actually work, not how we think they should work.

I anticipate there will be some people who do not like the message of this book. Those are people who like the myth, who believe the myth and who also often make money from the myth. My aim is not to convince these people. My aim is to ensure that the people who are suffering understand there is nothing wrong with them—the people who have blamed themselves, who have labelled themselves as failures, who have endlessly tried to be different but were unable to. This message is for you. The myth will continue to be generated because it holds a lot of power. Learn to ignore the myth. There is no point arguing with those who hold it dear. It is enough to simply live your own path and find your own truth. While the environment causes huge challenges for us when it comes to weight management, we can change how we respond to that environment. We can acknowledge the things we actually do, we can ignore unhelpful advice and we can be responsible for our health in a holistic manner. We don't have to be victims in this story.

I am a lot healthier now than I have been at other times in my life—even times when I was very thin. I am also happier. When I look at my health holistically I am in a really good position—I have amazing friendships, amazing family, inspired work, time for relaxation, plenty of laughter, spiritual fulfilment, drive and energy, peace of mind and contentment. If someone judges my health simply by the number of vegetables I eat a day or the number on the scales, they can go ahead. I know my health is doing better and better. I also know there will be times in my future where it slumps again. But that is the journey of health—it rides the ups and downs of life with me.

You can start your own journey by considering your health from a holistic perspective. There is an abundance of research identifying other factors that contribute to health other than weight. For example, having quality relationships is as important to your health as your body mass index and smoking status. Yet we rarely hear about this from our doctor or from health promotion activities. In fact, some researchers would even suggest that current data represents an underestimate of the importance of relationships on your health.

Altruism is also known from research to be health enhancing. Helping others and volunteering is a great option for health enhancement. Spending time outdoors is another contributing factor. Time admiring a beautiful sunset or walking through a rainforest or canoeing on a river can all have health benefits beyond any activity involved. Nature grounds us and tends to connect us with our spirituality. Even being able to see green space from our home and office windows is known to improve our wellbeing. Sleep and rest, time management, stress levels, meditation, spirituality and religion are all things that we know enhance our health.

As a result, we don't necessarily have to focus on our weight to focus on our health. It needs to be considered in a context of overall health and not be seen as the most important component. If you have spent years battling your weight, the best thing to do motivationally may be to focus on other health-enhancing factors for a while. For all we know, five minutes of deep breathing a day could influence your health as much as losing five kilograms. Or increasing time with people you love may have as much impact as losing ten kilograms. Spending time with people who judge and criticise you may be as bad as gaining weight. I'm not aware that research has even looked at these types of correlations. Even if your aim is to focus on your weight, don't try and do it in a void of other health-related activities. Consider a range of things that influence your wellbeing and they may reduce the possibility of health issues in relation to your weight. Overweight people can be healthy people, despite what we have been led to believe.

The easiest way for me to describe working with the motivation you have may be to describe how I have been doing that myself. The first thing that I acknowledge when it comes to my motivation is that it will fluctuate. My son, Evan, will be having major back surgery sometime in the next year. How he recovers from that surgery will have an influence on how I manage my health and wellbeing. For example, if it increases challenging behaviours again due to discomfort related to the surgery, I may go back to just surviving day to day. If that were to happen, I would probably start looking at harm-reduction strategies.

Harm reduction is a technique that developed in the field of drug and alcohol counselling. Motivationally, it is one of the toughest clinical fields to work in. Clients often aren't ready for abstinence. However, when you have a group of people who daily partake in dangerous activities, what do you do? The aim becomes to keep them and others around them safe. One day they may be ready for the idea of abstinence, but in the meantime the aim is to keep them alive, free from HIV or other diseases, out of jail and off the roads while under the influence, etc. Harm reduction is an approach designed to work with the motivation someone has at the time.

Harm-reduction strategies can be used for many different things though, including weight management. It could be as simple as drinking more water, eating more vegetables or walking only as far as the letterbox a couple of times a day. We use harm-reduction strategies for Evan, who has an obsession with cola. It is impossible to remove cola from his life. Where can you go outside of your home where there are no cola beverages? Nowhere! If he is unable to have cola, he becomes completely overwhelmed and anxious. We had to figure out a way to allow him to have cola but reduce the potential health concerns. As a result, we stock caffeine-free diet cola at home and pace out how often he can drink it. This is far from ideal—no one wants their child drinking this all the time, but he cannot calm himself down unless he has cola regularly. On a recent trip to the hospital, we walked past a café when he saw cola drinks displayed through the window. He literally laid himself down on the footpath in protest when we said he couldn't have one. Our lives can be very interesting at times! Motivationally, it is impossible for us to break this obsession and so we have had to find a way to live with it but reduce the potential harms of his consumption.

Harm reduction is a really good place to start when it comes to managing weight and health. The focus could be reducing weight gain rather than trying to lose weight. My one nutritional focus is to eat as many vegetables as I can. I have discovered I prefer to eat vegetables in the form of soup rather than eating salad or steamed vegetables. Soup has more flavour and feels heartier. I also like vegetable dips such as babaganoush, hummus and guacamole. Vegetables are not only full of nutrients and fibre, they reduce cholesterol. Rather than focusing too much on specific exercise sessions, I have tried to increase my daily movement around the workplace. I move with the ebb and flow of my motivation. My aim is to find a place within my motivation that sits between effortless and a daily battle. This is what that would look like in a diagram:

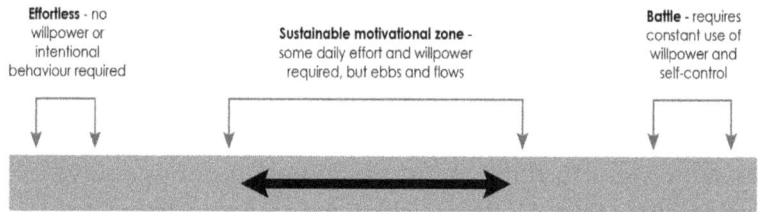

Note that there is still movement in my motivation at any one time. It could fluctuate throughout the day, from week to week, or I could have a bad period again where I stay down at the bottom end of the scale for several months. The aim though is not to go to either extreme on the scale to maintain my health as best I can without destroying my motivation. The extremes are where we sit when we either have false hope and think we can 'will' ourselves to change, or we feel completely hopeless and throw the towel in. Neither of these spaces actually coincide with weight management, but people who weight cycle jump from one end to the other.

By staying in the middle of the scale, it is possible to recognise that even when things are tough, you are still doing things to sustain your health. This helps remove the guilt of the fluctuations. One of the best things to do is to use a scale to demonstrate this process of fluctuation. Let's do an activity:

0   1   2   3   4   5   6   7   8   9   10
Effortless   Battle

Imagine 0 (zero) is doing nothing to take care of your health, and 10 (ten) is doing everything you can imagine to take care of your health.

Where do you think you currently sit on the scale? Circle the number.

I currently sit at a five.

Take a moment to think about the lowest number you've ever been on this scale. Circle the corresponding number.

I was at a two during my period of hopelessness.

What about the highest you've ever been on the scale? Circle it.

I have been as high as a seven.

For each of the numbers you circled, write the things you were doing at each of them. It is important to try to be very specific.

Life's too short to live without cheesecake

Examples of the things I was doing include the following:

2	5	7
I deliberately exercised about once a fortnight.	I deliberately exercised about three times a week.	I deliberately exercised about five times a week.
I ate whatever my mood dictated without restraint, but continued to eat vegetables every day and a healthy breakfast.	I increased my vegetable intake by making soup more often and made an effort to add more vegetables to sandwiches. I ate vegetable dips more often.	I rarely ate processed foods and was very focused on the nutritional content of the foods I ate.
I took medication for mental health.	I continued to take medication.	I did not require medication.
I did not see friends often—maybe once every four or five months.	I increased contact with friends—maybe monthly.	I had a monthly get-together pre-organised with friends.
I worked fulltime.	I reduced my working hours to four days a week to support my health.	I worked part-time—three days a week.
We did not receive support for Evan other than what we could pay for ourselves. This was not enough.	We received an increase in support connected to government funding for my son through the National Disability Insurance Scheme.	Support for Evan included his grandparents. His behaviour was much less challenging though and less support was required.
I was on the receiving end of very challenging behaviours from Evan, including a lot of violence.	Even's behaviours settled significantly. He was only occasionally violent and he easily de-escalated now.	Behavioural problems were present but minimal.
I did not meditate.	I meditated for about ten minutes three times a week.	I did not meditate.
I did not partake in yoga.	I partook in yoga twice a week for about ten minutes each session.	I partook in yoga four to five times a week for about half an hour each session.

I spent most of my time at home.	I increased outings and fun activities, such as going to restaurants, plays and festivals.	Evan was able to tolerate outings more easily, in particular activities with extended family.
I was exhausted all the time.	I felt rested and energised.	I felt exhaustion developing—it was sporadic in nature.
I prioritised sleep and rest over all other health needs.	I still prioritised sleep and rest.	I was sleeping poorly due to the ages of the children.
I felt hopeless and depressed.	I felt generally optimistic and looked forward to the future.	I felt mostly optimistic.
I didn't have the energy or desire to write.	Writing became a regular activity, which I was able to prioritise now because there was more help.	I hadn't discovered writing at this stage in my life.
I gained weight.	My weight was stable—there was a slight reduction over several months.	My weight was stable.

Life's too short to live without cheesecake

Now it's your turn:

Lowest number	Now	Highest number

Scaling activities clearly demonstrate that things fluctuate based on life circumstances. My health has drastically improved due to the increased help available through the National Disability Insurance Scheme, but this has had nothing to do with my personal effort and motivation. I also recognise that reducing my hours at work reduced the busyness in my life and improved my overall sense of wellbeing. Both these things supported my health. Neither of them involved setting a goal or creating a new habit.

This may be a part of a harsh reality. There may be things that could radically improve your health that you have no control over. For the sake of their health, many people would benefit from a reduction in their working hours. Most carers would be healthier if they had more help available to them. But both these things require structures outside of our control to support us. I therefore acknowledge some of the positive changes to my health have been driven and supported by other people.

We will need much more of this civic-minded thinking if we are to make headway when it comes to obesity. Let's imagine we lived in a world where we worked together as communities to reduce obesity:

- What would it be like if schools provided lunches to our children? Some countries already do this. Imagine how much pressure it would take off our parents. Imagine not running out of fruit at the end of the week? Or imagine never having that 'What do you want for lunch?' conversation again?

- What if employers also did this and had healthy snacks people could eat during the day? Imagine if you arrived at a meeting and there was a plate of freshly cut vegies, nuts and hummus to eat while you talked business. Would you eat more vegetables if you didn't have to think about it so much?

- And what if our employers gave us pedometers and actively encouraged breaks or short walks during the day? If it was recognised as an important part of the workday to move, what about going outside to stretch for fifteen minutes?

- Imagine if we created a culture where less was more when it came to kid's activities, homework and fundraising responsibilities? If we stopped treating childhood like a competition? If we recognised parents need to spend more downtime with their children rather than helping with homework sheets?

- What if we went back to children only having two birthday parties during their childhoods instead of ten? If mothers used their collective powers to reduce expectations placed on each other rather than increasing them? Would life be more fun with just a couple of pizzas and a store-bought cake?

- Imagine if we worked half an hour less a day. Or had more recreation leave time? If asking for a mental health day was normal and accepted as a good health practice? If we genuinely recognised as a community that rest is an essential part of health?

- What if there were no chocolates or soft drinks sold at sales counters? If instead they stocked items we actually need to be reminded about, such as toothpaste or sticky tape?

- If all restaurants and takeaways provided at least two serves of vegetables with each meal? If we didn't have to spend an extra seven dollars on 'steamed greens' to come with our steak and chips? If hamburger restaurants included a small salad as well as a small serve of fries with a standard meal deal?

- What if snacks were reduced in size by five to ten per cent? Do we really need muffins that big? Banana bread sliced that thickly? Coffees that size? We could still enjoy ourselves with a little bit less I'm sure!

- What if every council ensured we had safe, beautiful walking paths, outdoor concerts and art events, free gym equipment and swimming pools? Would we get out more?

If we were creative and determined as communities, there are many things we could develop that would reduce the reliance on our own personal 'motivation'. And that is where we need to start making more noise and taking more action—creating an environment that supports our health, rather than maintaining one that challenges it in such a debilitating way.

Another model that could be helpful to consider is called 'Small Changes' by James O. Hill. Small changes are an important part of ensuring weight management in the long term. This model specifies just how much small changes can make a difference. Hill and colleagues examined what is referred to as 'the energy gap' for different populations. They tracked the rate of weight gain in different communities and established just how much excess energy is required to support the noted rate of weight gain. The calculated what each individual would need to do to stop gaining weight, and the results were:

- Reduce their intake by three bites of food a day OR
- Increase activity by an additional 2,500 steps a day.

If we all did this every day, the obesity epidemic would literally stop in its tracks. It's quite compelling to consider. Of course, like many things that seem simple on paper, it could be much more complex than we think. But motivationally, this seems doable in comparison to other things I have read. Could you reduce your daily intake of food by three bites a day? This was calculated based on a hamburger, so it would have to be equivalent from a calories perspective. But three bites doesn't feel overwhelming, does it? The beauty of the theory is you don't need to change what you are eating at all, just alter how much. You could still have your beloved cheesecake! Or pasta, or beer, or potato crisps. So, it has great appeal. To come up with these recommendations, Hill and colleagues considered population-level statistics and variations in caloric requirements and metabolic rates. This figure would work for everyone! In fact, most people would actually lose a little bit of weight using this method.

I recently bought a fitness device that you wear like a watch. It has been quite an informative experience. I now know how little I move during my work week and how much I move on my weekends. It turns out that washing, cleaning, grocery shopping and the general day-to-day at home require a lot of steps! But my work days are another story! There are some days were I barely move from my desk. As a result of this information, I now consciously do a couple of walks during my workday. And while I have to remind myself, it feels easier than forcing myself to exercise. After all, I don't have to put on exercise clothes, I don't have to have a shower afterwards and I don't have to schedule a certain amount of time in my day. I also don't feel pressured or guilty. I just get up for five or ten minutes at a convenient time in my day and move. And I have discovered it is energising, great for clearing the mind, and also good for networking (because I inevitably run into people on my way)!

The Small Changes approach only requires one or the other to achieve the outcome. If you think you could manage to incorporate both, you would in fact lose weight. Keep in mind it would be very slow though! Years ago, my sister the dietitian told me the best rate of sustainable weight loss was approximately 0.5 kilograms a month. This is far slower than most people want to lose weight when they go on a 'diet'. The rate of weight loss is very important because it is indicative of being within the 'sustainable motivational zone'.

I have been slowly increasing my health-enhancing behaviours over the last eighteen months, and I have only just started to lose some weight! If my initial aim had been to lose weight, I would have given in by now! But my real aim has been to improve my health. I was gaining weight, so initially the changes would have slowly reduced the rate of weight gain, and then stabilised my weight. As the changes have increased, I have tipped to a point of slow weight loss. I have stayed within the sustainable motivational zone and I have maintained my motivation by knowing my health has improved, not by focusing on the number on the scales.

Having observed my motivation for some time, I know certain things about myself, and what I can change and what I can't:

- I can reduce my wine intake slightly by using a smaller glass and not having wine stored at the house (this inevitably means a few days a week without wine until

I get back to the shops).

- I am not going to get up at five am to exercise.
- I prefer vegetables in the form of soup or dip rather than salad.
- Sleep and rest remain my most important health activity—everything else falls apart when I am tired.
- I hate exercising when it is really hot—unless I am in the pool.
- Increasing my activity levels at work has been relatively easy with a little bit of conscious focus. It has brought more benefits than just my weight management.
- I love doing activities that give me a sense of peace and relaxation such as yoga and walking.
- I love to dance and forgot why I stopped listening to music. (I think it had something to do with the children and the amount of Wiggles music we listened to for years!)
- There are times when I love to cook and times when I don't. I never feel guilty about making my life easier when required.
- My caring responsibilities and my son's behaviours have a significant influence on my motivation. The more help I can get, the healthier I am from many perspectives.
- I am a giver more so than an achiever. My sense of purpose in life is linked to this and so it will always be my main motivational driver.

- Food is an important source of joy and celebration for me.

- I have the ability to use willpower regularly when I am not stressed or exhausted.

- Reducing how busy I am has increased my capacity to take care of my health.

- I don't necessarily need to exercise to increase my health-enhancing activity levels.

- My body is fine just as it is.

- I am still attractive to my husband despite any weight gain.

- I see myself as a work in progress.

- I have ditched any idea of perfectionism.

- My capacity to do health-related activities will fluctuate with things that are outside of my control.

- Writing on a regular basis is health enhancing for me.

- Life is too short to live without cheesecake.

The thing that is interesting about writing this list was how peaceful I felt as I wrote it. There's an ease to living life like this—taking the pressure off and understanding myself better. I no longer compare myself to other people in a negative way. I still have flashes of negative thinking about my weight that I have learnt to ignore. And I feel so free as a result of this self-acceptance.

CHAPTER 17

Questions you may have

'You spend most of your time living inside your head. Make sure it's a nice place to be.'

— Buddha

One of the struggles I had when writing this book was deciding how much information to put into it. My aim was to be informative without being overwhelming. This can be quite difficult when you've read a lot of research and have a lot of useful information to share. As a result, this book only touches the surface of many of the concepts discussed. I have tried to let the story provide the information more so than facts or figures. Inevitably though, this may leave people with some questions. I wanted to ensure I addressed at least some of the questions that may still be lingering.

1. **Should I weigh myself regularly?**

That may depend on who you are and the relationship you've had with your weight. If you've had a habit of feeling depressed when you get on the scales, or punishing yourself if it goes up slightly, I would suggest you need to stay away from weighing yourself for a while. On the other hand, it is also important to be informed about your weight and to keep an eye on what is happening with it.

You may need to train yourself over time to suspend judgement about the number on the scale. While there is research that suggests people who weigh themselves more often do better on diets, all these studies are short term and are based specifically on weight loss. The strategies I am recommending may have an impact on weight loss, but very slowly and in the longer term. Therefore, I suggest occasional weighing of yourself in order to be informed. This may be one of those times though when you use your intuition and think about what is best for you and where you are at right now.

2. **Would you recommend a personal fitness device such as a Fitbit?**

I personally found this very helpful. If you want to implement the Small Changes approach, you need to have some idea of your daily activity levels overall. But remember to use it as information and not to use it for punishment or guilt. The aim is to ditch those negative emotions and do things for yourself and your body with a sense of love and nurturing. You may need to use one for yourself and see how you feel. Some people have personalities that find it hard to use a device like this without feeling negative or frustrated. I have to admit that I completely avoid some of the settings on my device because I feel I am being nagged if I use them!

3. **What do you think of weight loss surgery?**

I completely understand the desire to use an option such as surgery if weight has been an ongoing issue over many years. However, this is a very serious decision with some potentially very serious consequences. It still requires considerable changes in behaviour, and therefore motivation is still going to be a component of long-term, sustainable change. This decision needs to be made in consultation with a healthcare provider who has experience in this field. You may have urgent health issues that need to be resolved as quickly as possible, and therefore surgery might be the least risky option. But these decisions are individual in nature and cannot be generalised.

4. **I am very concerned about a loved one's weight. How should I support them?**

You probably need to do the exact opposite of what you feel like doing. Remember that sensitivity to autonomy and nagging usually drive the person in the opposite direction. You need to give them love and understanding. Reading this book is a good starting point.

If the person is a child, ensure healthy meals and snacks are available but not to the exclusion of food they enjoy. Do activities as a family that are active and enjoyable. Do not nag about weight. Do not criticise what they eat. Do not even roll your eyes or sigh. They will sense all this judgement. Accept that this is a journey, and encourage a holistic approach to health that includes good sleep, time with friends and lots of laughter. Encourage a positive sense of body image. Research on adolescents showed that those who grew up with parents focusing on their weight ended up gaining more weight in the longer term. Be a positive role model regarding all these things yourself.

If the person you are concerned about is an adult, give them a copy of this book to read and the let them make their own decisions. Stay out of it. Only talk about it if they bring it up. Recognise the things they do for their health and do not criticise. Remember, people who love them unconditionally are as important to their health and wellbeing as their weight. Be one of those people. And don't assume they do less for their health than you. They may actually be doing better than you think!

5. **Should I do a weight loss program?**

While I have said 'no diets' in this book, I am not naïve enough to think people will actually follow this advice! There are lots of different types of programs out there and they are very tempting. One of the problems with weight loss programs is they aim for you to lose weight more rapidly than what really works with the sustainable motivational zone. Some have a personal consultant, which at least helps you to personalise your plan.

But be critical—are they focusing on setting goals and changing habits? These things are likely to be less successful than things that work with your personality and your values. Do they eliminate food or do they accommodate eating anything and balance it out? Do they have meal replacements or do they work with the food you actually eat every day?

While diets don't work, there may be parts of some programs that can be helpful for improving your knowledge and helping you to be more mindful about your eating and activity levels. Take the knowledge you have gained from this book and use your critical judgement skills. If you feel like you are being sold a fantasy, you probably are. Remember, slow weight loss is best, so even if you head down this path, pace it at a rate that provides a balance between your motivation and your desire to lose weight.

6. Should I go to a personal trainer?

My criteria for suggesting a personal trainer would be this—do you love to exercise? They could be helpful if you want to train for a triathlon, walk up Mount Kilimanjaro, cycle across Europe or complete some other major fitness challenge. But if you are like me and exercise is something you do when the weather feels right, you are in the mood or it helps you to relax, there is no point going to a personal trainer.

Your aim is to do things that you are motivationally driven towards naturally, not because someone is yelling instructions at you and pushing you beyond your comfort zone. If this is not your natural motivational state, personal trainers won't be something you can maintain in the longer term. They may also cause you irritation and possibly set off your need for autonomy. If you have ever been to a personal trainer and gone home to eat chocolate straight away, they are not for you!

7. Should I do assessments to find out more about my values profile and my personality?

You can certainly do this if you feel like it would be helpful. There are some online options. My recommendations would be to look for the 'Schwartz Values Assessment' and the 'Five Factor Model Personality Assessment'. There may be others, but I cannot vouch for their validity. Even doing the online assessments provide more of a guide than a true and accurate reflection. This is because, when the assessments are used under research conditions, they do more complex calculations than the ones that can be done for an online survey. However, I think it is quite useful to have some idea about how these motivational drivers work for you.

8. **I believe I have an over-eating disorder. Is this book still relevant to me?**

An eating disorder adds another layer of complexity to your motivational drivers and it is likely to be very deeply embedded. I am not an expert on eating disorders and so I would recommend you discuss the content with someone trained in this specialised field of practice. While the concepts discussed will still have some relevance, a disorder is often driven by something more complex.

Overall though, the points in this book remain relevant even with an eating disorder and can be helpful as part of a greater strategy.

9. **Isn't this just a bunch of excuses?**

There will be some people who see it this way. However, when working with people, I have always found excuses to be an indication of something deeper I need to explore. So yes, on the surface, people may seem to be making what appear to be excuses. Often though, the people making these excuses don't know why they are unmotivated or what is getting in the way. When people seem to be avoidant or making excuses, I see it as my role to explore deeper layers of the motivational profile to gain a greater understanding of why these excuses exist. The first place I generally start is with the concept of hope. Often, I find a story of repeated failure at weight management. Excuses to me just indicate a lack of working effectively with core motivators and set me on a path of discovery.

10. Do the concepts in this book relate to other aspects of motivation?

Yes. I did not learn about motivational principles from weight loss programs. I learnt about them from trying to help people do something other than smoke all day!

The principles are the same no matter what the motivational content. If you are struggling to study, it may be because you don't really value the outcome. If you are struggling to write a book, it may be because you have no hope that it will be published. If you are struggling to maintain a relationship, it may be because it impedes your personal autonomy. If you are struggling to cook, it may be because you actually hate doing it. If you don't want to take a promotion at work, it may be because your intuition is telling you it is not the right thing for you to do. As far as I can tell, all motivation makes sense and has a logic to it. Any motivational struggle you have can still be explored from the principles outlined in this book.

11. I want to feel good about my body as it is. How can I do that?

Don't expect miracles with something as complex as this. I still struggle too! What I do though is catch myself out when I am having a negative thought like 'I look fat in that photo'. The aim isn't to get rid of these thoughts, as they are bound to still come. The aim is to 'let them pass you by'. That is, notice the thought, but try not to react emotionally to it. They are going to come because we are constantly being marketed and groomed to think this way. Sometimes I say to myself, 'Be like

Teflon. Let it slide right off'. That will take practice though, possibly over a lifetime.

12. How can I raise children to think like this?

I recently read a story on social media about a woman who grew up without a set of scales in her house. She never questioned it and it was only as an adult she discovered her mother had done this deliberately. Health discussions never focused on weight, they always focused on broad overall concepts. She was protecting her children from being obsessed with weight. I thought this was quite brilliant! The best thing overall though is to live the reality of these messages as an entire family. I never talk negatively about my body or envy someone else's body in front on my family (I try not to do it at all but am particularly vigilant in front of my children). There are no foods that are banned from my house. We watch television shows with people of all diversities, including people with disabilities, from different cultures, with different types of beauty and different sexualities. We prioritise rest and do not over-schedule our lives. We have good sleeping patterns. We celebrate our individuality, good and bad. There is no recipe. But you can't fake this. You can't say you love your body as it is and then get a boob job. You can't hide your body under layers of clothes and claim to be perfectly happy. Kids absorb the entire story, not just what is coming out of your mouth. If you are trying to fake it, they will know whether you say it or not. So, the primary aim is to live it yourself.

13. Short-term motivation versus long-term gain

Things that are immediate have a greater influence on our motivation than something that has the potential for long-term gain. People can endlessly convince themselves to start their diet next week, to quit smoking in the New Year, to save money *after* they've purchased this very expensive handbag. We need to understand this and have some acceptance of it. Use willpower when you have it and know there will be times when it is not strong enough to cope with this immediate temptation.

14. Do you hate skinny fit people?

Not at all. They are just different. The only thing I hate is when skinny fit people are held up as being more successful than other people in the community. That is something we can all influence and, if we work together as a community, we can reduce this community belief. The message is causing the problems, not the people who love fitness and nutrition. Body-shaming comes from many people in many circumstances. The first step is to not shame our own bodies. Once we have done that, we can stop adding shame to other people's bodies. That is not the job of skinny people, it is the job of us all.

15. A small group of people do lose a lot of weight through diets and keep it off. Who are these people?

While I don't know this answer for sure, my guess would be these are the people who have lost weight in line with their natural motivators. This makes the maintenance stage possible for them when the rest of us would struggle. They may also have been the people who have lost it slowly. I think there is another group, though, who get an awful lot of attention if they gain or lose weight and this influences how their motivation works. Anyone who has a public profile and loses weight is likely to receive gains from the weight loss and perhaps better job security as a result. This will influence their ability to keep it off more effectively.

16. Is the original Motivation to Create Change (MCC) Theory still relevant?

This was the tool I originally came up with to describe motivational concepts to my colleagues. Here it is again:

1. People will only be motivated if they are interested in the change.

2. People will only be motivated if they have hope that the change is possible.

3. People will only be motivated if they have a clear vision of what this change looks like.

4. People will only be motivated if they believe they have the capacity to create the change.

5. People will only be motivated if they value the difference the change will make to their lives.

6. People will only be motivated if their intuition tells them this change feels right, right now.

7. People will only be motivated if they feel in control of the process to create the change.

8. People will only be motivated if they are prepared to tolerate the discomfort the change process will bring.

It still has relevance and, as you can see, the things in the theory have all been described at some point in the book. However, it is only a tool and is not a complete guide to motivation. I do have colleagues who use the theory when working with their clients and say it is extremely useful. It enables them to have a more in-depth discussion with their clients about motivation and where barriers may be present.

It also offers a quick and simple means of looking at your motivation for any issue. I used it when I was trying to figure out why I wasn't motivated to write academic articles! I rated each item of the MCC Theory out of ten and realised I didn't really value the outcome and I was only interested because other people thought it would be good for me to do! You can use it in a similar way if you feel 'stuck' when it comes to your motivation.

17. **What now?**

Don't rush into anything. Don't try and turn this into the latest 'fad'. Don't do anything except absorb and reflect on the information in this book. How do you see the evidence of the ideas in your own life? In others? Remember you are supposed to be working with who you are, not launching into another set of goals and new habits. This will take time and it will take some trial and error. You will start to notice the things that don't work first. You may start to notice that when your friend suggests a new exercise fad, your mind thinks 'no thanks'. Your mind is telling you where your motivation lies for that activity. If you have to convince yourself to give it a try, it's not for you. You will notice that no matter how often you have tried to stop, ice-cream from your favourite parlour is pure joy, and something you look forward to or see as a reward. Keep it. It has a degree of meaning. You will notice that straight after work is the hardest time to even contemplate exercise. You may be too exhausted or too busy focusing on the next set of jobs that have to be done.

Eventually you will also start to notice when you naturally do things that are good for your health. You will notice you really enjoy a piece of fruit with breakfast. You will notice that a walk in the local park that is shady and quiet is incredibly enjoyable on a weekend. You will notice that cooking with your kids involved makes it feel like family time rather than a chore. You will start to notice all the little nuances that are naturally occurring and they will start to make more sense to you. Once you have a better sense of yourself, you are in a better place to consider changes—small, deliberate changes that work for you and your life that are easily absorbed and have no sense of battle attached to them.

18. **Where can I read more?**

I have deliberately written this book for the general community. As a result, I have mentioned research without providing too much detail. If, however, you are interested in exploring the detail of the research and increasing your understanding from an evidence-based perspective, I have included a bibliography at the end of the book.

19. **I work with people in the health industry and would like to learn how to work with people and their motivation in the way discussed in this book. How can I learn more?**

I do post videos, blogs and provide webinars on various topics related to motivation. At times, I also present workshops or lectures. The best way to keep up to date with opportunities is to follow my social media accounts or to go to the website **www.josherring.com**.

CHAPTER 18

Tess and the dress

'The mind, once stretched by a new idea, can never return to its former dimensions'

— Ralph Waldo Emerson

Tess did in fact go and buy a bigger dress. But only after I got her to read the first three draft chapters of this book. If no one else reads it, at least I have achieved my initial aim!

The message in this book isn't necessarily easy to absorb or accept. In fact, for many it may be quite confronting. In essence, I am saying we as individuals may well continue to be overweight and obese. That is not what people want to hear and, believe me, it is not a message I necessarily want to deliver. But I believe we are facing a scenario in which human beings can only do so much as individuals to manage this problem. My aim therefore is to help people to do what they can within their individual circumstances and capacity. The situation is challenging, but it is not hopeless. Just because we may not be able to lose great amounts of weight does not mean we can't considerably improve our health outcomes, but we will need to start measuring this in more holistic ways than by the body mass index.

Part of the problem has been the way we as individuals and communities have responded to the problem. We have increased knowledge and we have increased intention, but we have not increased positive outcomes. This unfortunately has an impact on the motivation of individuals, leading to a dynamic of self-blame and hopelessness. I believe this has significantly added to the overall problem. However, as individuals we can choose to respond to this challenge differently. We can stop focusing on the number on the scale and start focusing on broader health. We can stop listening to unhelpful messages and start pushing for new ones. We can recognise all the little things we do for our health and start gradually building on them in alignment with our motivation. And we can stop looking at body shapes as signs of success or failure and be grateful for the bodies we have.

While it is tempting to throw in the towel on weight management (and I understand how that happens), we cannot stay in a space of hopeless despair. We must take care of our health, the health of our loved ones and our communities. We just have been looking for the answer to the problem in the wrong location. We have tried to rely on individual human motivation and denial to resolve the issue. But human beings are just human beings in the context they find themselves. Their normal motivation has many influences, some that they can control and some that they cannot. If we refocus our attention, our research, our demands and our efforts, it is quite possible we can successfully meet the challenge of obesity. But it won't be in the form of a meal replacement or an exercise program. It will be in the form of a committed community and a new social environment.

This new world needs to have some specific elements to help us create the solutions for obesity:

1. We need to stop blaming and judging individuals.

2. We need to broaden our perspective of health.

3. We need to accept all bodies in a positive manner.

4. We need to recognise the efforts of individuals to take care of their health.

5. We need to stop providing generalised information and start targeting individuals in their personal circumstances.

6. We need to reduce endless temptations.

7. We need to make healthy food easy and accessible.

8. We need to reorganise schools and workplaces to embrace movement.

9. We need to provide fun, interesting, free options for movement in our community spaces.

10. We need to refocus our research efforts on environmentally based interventions.

11. We need to find options through research for individuals with genetically based weight gain.

12. We need to resolve issues related to weight gain from medications and other medical interventions.

13. We need to reduce stress and increase time for health activities.

14. We need to skill up health professionals in normal human motivation and working with it more effectively.

15. We need to stop telling people to get motivated.

16. We need to stop putting bouncy, ponytail girls on the television as 'inspiration'.

We need to create a world like Whole Foods Markets®. This is a supermarket chain in the United States that I came across when travelling. It holds a particular philosophy, and everything in the store is established to make it easy for consumers to stick to this philosophy. The products in the store all meet a set of standards. They are organic, ethically produced and environmentally sustainable. Rather than expecting their customers to do all the work, they have done it for us. Every item you buy there has been tested to meet the ethics of the organisation. This covers not only food items but toiletries, cleaning products, cosmetics, etc., too. Of course, as a result, this supermarket is quite expensive. And yet it is easy. So easy, my individual human motivation is not required. All I have to do is show up and shop.

They also have another amazing section in their supermarkets where you can purchase fresh and healthy meals. They have freshly cooked fish, stir-fries, noodles, soups, salads, baked vegetables, rice, fruit and anything else you could want for a healthy meal. You just pick up their environmentally friendly containers and fill them up with as much or as little as you like. The cost is based on weight, so you can buy enough for a family meal or just one serve. This was so handy while we travelled. My fussy-eating daughter could find something she liked, my husband could eat something full of chilli, and I could keep it simple with steamed fish and vegetables to balance out all the fast food you inevitably eat on a trip. I thought this was the most amazing idea and how it would enable all working parents to pull in on their way home from work to pick something up for dinner without worrying if it is healthy or not.

If we could think more like Whole Foods Markets® in the creating of our communities, I think we would be on the road to success. Sitting around and waiting for people to 'get motivated' hasn't worked, so we need to take that out of the equation. We need to make this as easy as we can. That's why schools providing lunch and workplaces having platters of dip and vegies would help. People wouldn't have to think about it—it would just be a part of the social structure. Maybe we should be moving the students around to different locations for different classes rather than having them sit all day. Free kid-friendly dance classes at the local park once a week might also help. But we need to draw people out and make it simple. Exhausted, overwhelmed, busy people are going to be fat. We can spend our energy blaming them or we can spend our energy helping them.

Life's not just too short to live without cheesecake. It's too short to battle ourselves. It's too short to feel guilty every time we eat food. It's too short to despise the bodies we have. It's too short to count calories every day. It's too short to do things we hate. The longest life isn't necessarily the best life, not if it doesn't include cheesecake.

Health is a story with many chapters. There will be chapters where health is easy and chapters where it seems hard to attain. When I was feeling hopeless, I went to my GP for a check-up. She asked if I was doing any exercise, and I was embarrassed to admit that I was only walking the dog about once a week. I expected to hear the usual, 'You really need to do a bit more than that'. Instead she said, 'That's a lot more than some people do.' I could have hugged her. There was no lecture, there was no judgement and there was no guilt. She said the perfect thing at the perfect time for my motivation. She knew me well enough to know I was doing the best I could. And I think that was really important. It wasn't a one-off consultation in which a health practitioner flippantly listed off the 'standard advice'. It was a relationship. She knew me. She knew my kids. She knew my husband. She knew my circumstances. And she knew that this was a moment in time of a much bigger health story. And as a result, she was genuinely helpful. And I loved her for it.

The story of health is important and necessary to understand, but the current point in the story is just that. It's is not the beginning and it is not the end. Real stories are not linear. They don't go from A to B without drama, without courage, without despair. Most of us still have years of a story to create, and we can choose how the next chapters look. We can choose to step up to the challenge of our health, we can choose passion and energy, and we can choose acceptance of ourselves. We can choose to change our world and make it easier for everyone to manage their weight.

Environmental factors have a huge impact in all areas of health and we have known about this for decades. We know a poorer socioeconomic status is linked to smoking and drug use. We know that access to education dramatically improves health outcomes. We know that trauma leads to mental illness. We know that carers have poorer overall health. We know that lonely people die younger. And we know that living in a Western culture with access to plentiful food and sedentary lifestyles leads to steady weight gain over a person's lifetime. We can't keep blaming the individuals in these scenarios. It's as helpful as walking into war-torn Syria with a book called 'How to find happiness in all situations'. Positive thinking and gratitude aren't going to be enough. And neither is 'set a goal and stick to it' when it comes to obesity. It doesn't work, and it never has.

There is a doctor at my local hospital doing research on the impact of gut bacteria on weight. The research involves a faecal transplant from a slim person and putting it into an overweight person (yes, it is as gross as it sounds). But they had amazing results with this technique in mice and their first trial on a human (who was another doctor) resulted in the person losing thirty kilograms without changing eating or exercise habits. Imagine if obesity came down to something like gut bacteria? There is hope, but we've been looking for it in the wrong places. Human beings are delightfully imperfect creatures. And that is exactly how we are meant to be. We wouldn't want it any other way when we think about it.

If the most interesting thing we achieve in life is thinness, would that be enough? Would we feel like the essence of our soul has been expressed? Would we have left a mark on the world that no one can remove? Would we have lived joyfully and passionately? The healthiest people I know live their life authentically, driven by the things they care deeply about, excited to be themselves and living their own path. Let's be that type of healthy. It may not get us on the cover of a magazine when we are sixty, but who the hell cares? Our soul will sing while our arse wobbles, and what a fabulous sight that would be!

Acknowledgements

A book is never completed alone, and there have been many people who have helped me along the way.

Karen Metcalfe reviewed my initial drafts and always made me feel like an amazing writer. She found the perfect balance of critique mixed with kindness, and her encouragement and love through the journey was a huge blessing.

Mary Anne Anderson not only inspired me to live an authentic life but had some incredibly useful feedback to polish the book in a way I would never have achieved alone.

A number of other people also took the time to read some of the initial drafts. Peter, Tess, Amanda, Carrie, Narelle—if you hadn't supported the first few chapters, the book would never have been completed.

Amanda Newton dragged me out of moments of self-doubt and was always on hand when I needed reminding that the book had an important message. I also thank her for the photography and graphic design work in the book.

There are quite a number of people who allowed me to share their personal stories. Thank you for allowing me to bring life to the book by sharing real-life struggles. Peter was particularly generous in allowing me to divulge his personal habits and eccentricities!

To all the researchers whose valued work I've mentioned in this book: while I discovered I was not an academic, I am so grateful to those who spend their lives answering questions through research. It can be slow, tedious, detailed work and there is often little recognition for the work you do. But without your collective efforts, we would continue to struggle with the big questions about life.

To all the clients I worked with as a clinician in mental health services: it was your stories that taught me to see the world with new eyes, to question and to discover.

To my children, Evan and Maya, who not only inspire me every day but fill the house with laughter and love.

And most importantly, again to my husband Peter, who lived the journey of hopelessness and despair with me, held me when the tears came, believed in my ideas and my writing, and always told me I was beautiful no matter what I weighed. You said I could write a book, and well, here we are...

Interest Cards by Jo Sherring

Want to discover your strong interests and passions in life?

Interest Cards help you to reflect on the things that bring you energy, joy and fulfilment.

These cards can be used by individuals for personal reflection or by people wanting to facilitate discussions on interests with others.

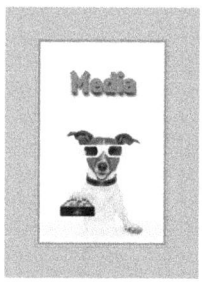 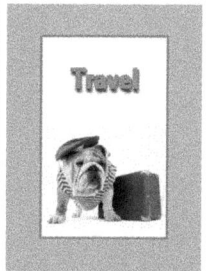
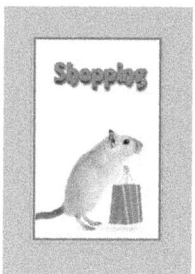 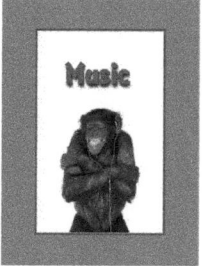

The box contains

- 50 full colour interest cards with humorous animal photos
- 15 coloured discussion/reflection cards.

See www.josherring.com for more information and purchase details.

Bibliography

Bardi, A, Buchanan, KE, Goodwin, R, Slabu, L & Robinson, M 2014, 'Value stability and change during self-chosen life transitions: Self-selection versus socialization effects', *Journal of Personality and Social Psychology*, vol. 106, no. 1, pp. 131–147.

Bardi, A & Goodwin, R 2011, 'The dual route to value change: Individual processes and cultural moderators', *Journal of Cross-Cultural Psychology*, vol. 42, no.2, pp. 271–287.

Bardi, A, Lee, JA, Hofmann-Towfigh, N, & Soutar, G 2009, 'The structure of intraindividual value change', *Journal of Personality and Social Psychology*, vol. 97, no. 5, pp. 913–929.

Bardi, A & Schwartz, SH 2003, 'Values and behaviour: Strength and structure of relations', *Personality and Social Psychology Bulletin'*, vol. 29, no.10, pp. 1207–1220.

Calogero, RM, Bardi, A & Sutton, RM 2009, 'A need basis for values. Associations between the need for cognitive closure and value priorities', *Personality and Individual Differences*, vol. 46, no.2, pp. 154–159.

Cole, DN & Hall, TE 2010, 'Experiencing the restorative components of wilderness environments: Does congestion interfere and does length of exposure matter?', *Environment and Behavior*, vol. 42, no. 6, pp. 806–823.

Deci, EL, Koestner, R & Ryan, RM 1999, 'A meta-analytic review of experiments examining the effects of extrinsic rewards on intrinsic motivation', *Psychological Bulletin*, vol. 125, no. 6, pp. 627–668.

Deci, EL & Ryan, RM (eds.) 2002, *Handbook of Self-Determination Research*, The University of Rochester Press, Rochester, NY.

De Hoog, N, Stroebe, W & de Wit, JBF 2005, 'The impact of fear appeals on processing and acceptance of action recommendations', *Personality and Social Psychology Bulletin*, vol. 31, no. 1, pp. 24–33.

de Lorgeril, M, Salen, P, Paillard, F, Laporte, F, Boucher, F & de Leiris, J 2002, 'Mediterranean diet and the French paradox: Two distinct biogeographic concepts for one consolidated scientific theory on the role of nutrition in coronary heart disease', *Cardiovascular Research*, vol. 54, no.3, pp. 503–515.

Elfhag, K & Rossner, S 2005, 'Who succeeds in maintaining weight loss? A conceptual review of factors associated with weight loss maintenance and weight regain', *Obesity reviews*, vol. 6, no.1, pp. 67–85.

Epel, E, Lapidus, R, McEwan, B & Brownell, K 2001, 'Stress may add bite to appetite in women: A laboratory study of stress-induced cortisol and eating behavior', *Psychoneuroendocrinology*, vol. 26, no.1, pp. 37–49.

Fischer, R & Schwartz, S 2011, 'Whence differences in value priorities?: Individual, cultural, or artifactual sources', *Journal of Cross-Cultural Psychology*, vol. 42, no. 7, pp. 1127–1144.

Goodwin, R, Polek, E & Bardi, A 2012, 'The temporal reciprocity of values and beliefs: A longitudinal study within a major life transition', *European Journal of Personality*, vol. 26, no. 3, pp. 360–370.

Haines, J, Neumark-Sztainer, D, Wall, M & Story, M 2007, 'Personal, behavioral, and environmental risk and protective factors for adolescent overweight', *Obesity*, vol. 15, no. 11, pp. 2748–2760.

Hill, JO 2009, 'Can a small-changes approach help address the obesity epidemic? A report of the Joint Task Force of the American Society for Nutrition, Institute of Food Technologists, and International Food Information Council', *American Journal of Clinical Nutrition*, vol. 89, no.2, pp. 477–484.

Hill, JO, Peters, JC & Wyatt, HR 2009, 'Using the Energy Gap to address obesity: A commentary', *Journal of American Dietetic Association*, vol. 109, no. 11, pp. 1848–1853.

Hill, JO, Wyatt, HR & Melanson, EL 2000, 'Genetic and environmental contributions to obesity', *Medical Clinics of North America*, vol. 84, no. 2, pp. 333–346.

Hill, JO, Wyatt, HR, Reed, GW & Peters, JC 2003, 'Obesity and the environment: Where do we go from here?', *Science*, vol. 299, no. 5608, pp. 853–855.

Hofmann, W, Vohs, KD & Baumeister, RF 2012, 'What people desire, feel conflicted about, and try to resist in everyday life', *Psychological Science*, vol. 23, no. 6, pp. 582–588.

Holt-Lunstad, J, Smith, TB & Layton, JB 2010, 'Social relationships and mortality risk: A meta-analytic review', PLoS

Med 7(7):e1000316. https://doi.org/10.1371/journal.pmed.1000316.

Jeffery, RW, French, SA, Raether, C & Baxter, JE 1994, 'An environmental intervention to increase fruit and salad purchases in a cafeteria', *Preventive Medicine*, vol. 23, no.6, pp.788–792.

Job, V, Bernecker, K, Miketta, S & Friese, M 2015, 'Implicit theories about willpower predict the activation of a rest goal following self-control exertion', *Journal of Personality and Social Psychology*, vol. 109, no. 4, pp. 694–706.

Lally, P & Gardner, B 2011, 'Promoting habit formation', *Health Psychology Review,* vol. 7, suppl. 1, pp. S137–S158, DOI: 10.1080/17437199.2011.603640

Lally, P, Wardle, J & Gardner, B 2011, 'Experiences of habit formation: A qualitative study', *Psychology, Health & Medicine*, vol. 16, no. 4, pp. 484–489.

Larsen, JK, Geenen, R, Maas, C, de Wit, P, van Antwerpen, T, Brand, N & van Ramshorst, B 2004, 'Personality as a predictor of weight loss maintenance after surgery for morbid obesity', *Obesity Research*, vol. 12, no. 11, pp. 1828–1834.

Linde, JA, Jeffery, RW, French, SA, Pronk, NP & Boyle, RG 2005, 'Self-weighing in weight gain prevention and weight loss trials', *Annals of Behavioral Medicine*, vol. 30, no. 3, pp.210–216.

Lyubomirsky, S 2010, 'Hedonic Adaptation to positive and negative experiences', in Folkman, S (ed.), *The Oxford Handbook of Stress, Health and Coping*, Oxford University Press, New York, pp. 200–224.

Lyubomirsky, S, Sheldon, KM & Schkade, D 2005, 'Pursuing happiness. The architecture of sustainable change', *Review of General Psychology*, vol. 9, no. 2, pp.111–131.

Mann, T, Tomiyama, AJ, Westling, E, Lew, AM, Samuels, B & Chatman, J 2007, 'Medicare's search for effective obesity treatments: Diets are not the answer', *American Psychologist*, vol. 62, no. 3, pp. 220–233.

McDermott, D & Snyder, CR 1999, *Making Hope Happen: A workbook for turning possibilities into reality*, New Harbinger Publications Inc., Oakland, CA.

Meliema, A & Bassili, JN, 1995, 'On the relationship between attitudes and values: Exploring the moderating effects of self-monitoring and self-monitoring schematicity', *Personality and Social Psychology Bulletin*, vol. 21, no.9, pp. 885–892.

Neal, DT, Wood, W & Drolet, A 2013, 'How do people adhere to goals when willpower is low? The profits (and pitfalls) of strong habits', *Journal of Personality and Social Psychology*, vol. 104, no. 6, pp. 959–975.

Newman, E, O'Connor, DB & Conner, M 2007, 'Daily hassles and eating behaviour: The role of cortisol reactivity status', *Psychoneuroendocrinology*, vol. 32, no. 2, pp.125–132.

Ng, DM & Jeffery, RW 2003, 'Relationships between perceived stress and health behaviors in a sample of working adults', *Health Psychology*, vol. 22, no. 6, pp. 638–642.

Nix, GA, Ryan, RM, Manly, JB & Deci, EL 1999, 'Revitalization through self-regulation: The effects of autonomous and controlled motivation on happiness and vitality', *Journal of*

Experimental Social Psychology, vol. 35, no. 3, pp. 266–284.

Oaten, M & Cheng, K 2005, 'Academic examination stress impairs self-control', *Journal of social and clinical psychology*, vol. 24, no. 2, pp.254–279.

O'Connor, DB, Jones, F, Conner, M, McMillan, B & Ferguson, E 2008, 'Effects of daily hassles and eating style on eating behavior', *Health Psychology*, vol. 27, no. 1, suppl., pp. S20–S31.

Parks-Leduc, L, Feldman, G & Bardi, A 2014, 'Personality traits and personal values: A meta-analysis', *Personality and Social Psychology Review*, vol. 19, no. 1, pp. 3–29, https://doi.org/10.1177/1088868314538548.

Quick, V, Wall, M, Larson, N, Haines, J & Neumark-Sztainer, D 2013, 'Personal, behavioral and socio-environmental predictors of overweight incidence in young adults: 10-yr longitudinal findings', *International Journal of Behavioral Nutrition and Physical Activity*, vol. 10, no. 37, https://doi.org/10.1186/1479-5868-10-37.

Roccas, S, Sagiv, L, Schwartz, SH & Knafo, A 2002, 'The big five personality factors and personal values', *Personality and Social Psychology Bulletin*, vol. 28, no. 6, pp. 789–801.

Rohan, MJ 2000, 'A rose by any name? The values construct', *Personality and Social Psychology Review*, vol. 4, no.3, pp. 255–277.

Rokeach, M 1971, 'Long-range experimental modification of values, attitudes and behavior', *American Psychologist*, vol. 26, no. 5, pp.453–459.

Rozin, P, Fischler, C, Imada, S, Sarubin, A & Wrzesniewski, A 1999, 'Attitudes to food and the role of food in life in the U.S.A., Japan, Flemish Belgium and France: Possible implications for the diet-health debate', *Appetite*, vol. 33, no.2, pp. 163–180.

Schultz, W 2002, 'Getting formal with dopamine and reward', *Neuron*, vol. 36, no.2, pp. 241–263.

Schultz, W 2013, 'Updating dopamine reward signals', *Current Opinion in Neurobiology*, vol. 23, no. 2, pp. 229–238.

Schwartz, SH 2006, *Basic human values: Theory, methods and applications*, http://citeseerx.ist.psu.edu/viewdoc/download?doi=10.1.1.510.6950&rep=rep1&type=pdf.

Schwartz, SH & Bardi, A 2001, 'Value hierarchies across cultures: Taking a similarities perspective', *Journal of Cross-Cultural Psychology*, vol. 32, no. 3, pp. 268–290.

Schwartz, SH, Cieciuch, J, Vecchione, M, Davidov, E, Fischer, R, Beierlein, Ramos, A, Verkasalo, M, Lönnqvist, J-E, Demirutku, K, Dirilen-Gumus, O & Konty, M 2012, 'Refining the theory of basic individual values', *Journal of Personality and Social Psychology*, vol. 103, no. 4, pp. 663–688.

Shilts, MK, Horowitz, M & Townsend, MS 2004, 'Goal setting as a strategy for dietary and physical activity behavior change: A review of the literature', *American Journal of Health Promotion*, vol. 19, no. 2, pp. 81–93.

Snyder, CR 1994, *The Psychology of Hope: You can get there from here*, Free Press, New York.

Snyder, CR (ed.) 2000, *Handbook of Hope: Theory, Measures and Applications*, Academic Press, San Diego.

Snyder, LB, Hamilton, MA, Mitchell, EW, Kiwanuka-Tondo, J, Fleming-Milici, F & Proctor, D 2004, 'A meta-analysis of the effect of mediated health communication campaigns on behavior change in the United States', *Journal of Health Communication*, vol. 9, suppl. 1, pp. 71–96.

Sullivan, S, Cloninger, CR, Przybeck, TR & Klein, S 2007, 'Personality characteristics in obesity and relationship with successful weight loss', *International Journal of Obesity*, vol. 31, no.4, pp. 669–674.

Sutin, AR, Ferucci, L, Zonderman, AB & Terracciano, A 2011, 'Personality and obesity across the adult lifespan', *Journal of Personality and Social Psychology*, vol. 101, no. 3, pp. 579–592.

Teixeira, PJ, Silva, MN, Mata, J, Palmeira, AL & Markland, D 2012, 'Motivation, self-determination, and long-term weight control', *International Journal of Behavioral Nutrition and Physical Activity*, vol. 9, no. 22, https://doi.org/10.1186/1479-5868-9-22.

Thow, AM, Downs, S & Jan, S 2014, 'A systematic review of the effectiveness of food taxes and subsidies to improve diets: Understanding the recent evidence', *Nutrition Reviews*, vol. 72, no. 9, pp. 551–565.

van't Riet, J, Sijtsema, SJ, Dagevos, H & De Bruijn, GJ 2011, 'The importance of habits in eating behaviour: An overview and recommendations for future research', *Appetite*, vol. 57, no. 3, pp. 585–596.

Verhoeven, AA, Adriaanse, MA, Evers, C & de Ridder, DT 2012, 'The power of habits: Unhealthy snacking behaviour is primarily predicted by habit strength', *British Journal of Health Psychology*, vol. 17, no. 4, pp. 758–770.

Volkow, ND, Wang, GJ, Maynard, L, Jayne, M, Fowler, JS, Zhu, W, Logan, J, Gatley, SJ, Ding, YS, Wong, C & Pappas, N 2003, 'Brain dopamine is associated with eating behaviours in humans', *International Journal of Eating Disorders*, vol. 33, no. 2, pp. 136–142, DOI:10.1002/eat.10118.

Webb, TL, Sheeran, P & Luszczynska, A 2009, 'Planning to break unwanted habits: Habit strength moderates implementation intention effects on behaviour change', *British Journal of Social Psychology*, vol. 48, pp. 507–523.

Williams, GC, Grow, VM, Freedman, ZR, Ryan, RM & Deci, EL 1996, 'Motivational predictors of weight loss and weight-loss maintenance', *Journal of personality and social psychology*, vol. 70, no. 1, pp. 115–126.

Worsley, A 2002, 'Nutrition knowledge and food consumption: Can nutrition knowledge change food behaviour?', *Asia Pacific Journal of Clinical Nutrition*, vol. 11, Suppl. 3, pp. S579–S585.

Printed in Australia
AUOW01n1055030818
301014AU00005B/5